Public Mental Health Marketing: Developing a Consumer Attitude

Public Mental Health Marketing: Developing a Consumer Attitude

Donald R. Self, DBA
Editor

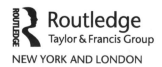

Routledge
Taylor & Francis Group

NEW YORK AND LONDON

Public Mental Health Marketing: Developing a Consumer Attitude has also been published as *Journal of Nonprofit & Public Sector Marketing,* Volume 1, Numbers 2/3 1993.

First published by 1993
The Haworth Press, Inc., 10 Alice Street, Binghamton, NY 13904-1580 USA

Published 2012 by Routledge

Routledge   Routledge
Taylor & Francis Group   Taylor & Francis Group
711 Third Avenue   2 Park Square, Milton Park, Abingdon,
New York, NY 10017   Oxfordshire OX14 4RN

First issued in paperback 2016

Routledge is an imprint of the Taylor and Francis Group, an informa business

Library of Congress Cataloging-in-Publication Data

Public mental health marketing : developing a consumer attitude / Donald R. Self, editor.
   p. cm.
   Published also as v. 1, no. 2/3 (1993) of the Journal of nonprofit & public sector marketing.
   ISBN 1-56024-189-6 (acid free paper)
   1. Mental health promotion – United States. 2. Mental health services – United States – Marketing. I. Self, Donald R.
RA790.53.P83 1990
362.2'068'8 – dc20   91-41001
                                        CIP

ISBN 13: 978-1-138-98423-3 (pbk)
ISBN 13: 978-1-56024-189-8 (hbk)

Public Mental Health Marketing: Developing a Consumer Attitude

Public Mental Health Marketing: Developing a Consumer Attitude

CONTENTS

ABOUT THE EDITOR

Donald R. Self, DBA, is Professor of Marketing at Auburn University, Montgomery, Alabama. An active health care and wellness consultant, Dr. Self has worked with various health care facilities, state and national agencies, and trade associations. He is a principal in Alabama Health Marketing Consultants and has published widely in professional journals, including *Health Marketing Quarterly, Journal of Marketing for Mental Health, Journal of Hospital Marketing,* and *Journal of Professional Services Marketing.* Dr. Self is also the editor of *Alcoholism Treatment Marketing: Beyond T.V. Ads and Speeches* (The Haworth Press, Inc., 1989) and co-editor of *Marketing for Health and Wellness Programs* (The Haworth Press, Inc., 1990).

Preface

This volume concludes a trilogy effort (Self 1989, Self and Busbin 1990) on the part of this editor and student of health care marketing into several related areas. During the mid and late 1980s, we were blessed with several opportunities to do research in the related areas of alcoholism treatment marketing, wellness program marketing, and the marketing of mental illness rehabilitation. The interrelationship between these three elements of health care marketing is extremely strong in that each involves a high level of involvement of the brain.

Of these three, this current volume was the most difficult. The status of Mental Health treatment and marketing, especially in the governmental and nonprofit sectors of the economy is truly that of a "growth industry poised on disaster." The growth element stems from recent research identifying specific areas of the brain as being responsible for mental wellness or mental illness. The disaster element is based on the continual fights for and periodic reductions in funding for mental health activities.

For those who would reallocate funds away from mental health activities, the stakes are high. In 1980 expenditures for mental health services were estimated at $20 billion (Frank and Kamlet). However, mental illness indirectly cost the country another $20 billion in lost time, total disability and premature death (Presidents Commission Vol. II, p. 530). In addition to the funding crisis in which all governmental agencies find themselves in 1993, the mental health field contains several challenges for managers and marketers.

For those who perform the social marketing tasks which will be required to bring the mentally recovering population back into society, facing the economic realities, the stakes are even higher. Much of the progress which has been made during the last decades is "at risk." Additionally, major problems remain beyond funding including the prevalence of stigmatic perceptions among the general public, the media, and potential employers; difficulty in finding housing and economic necessities during the readjustment stage; and difficulties which inevitably arise during the readjustment stage.

The reduction of stigma among various publics may be the one single area in which marketers can aid in the enhancement of the Public Mental Health system. This has been a major goal of the National Alliance of Mentally Ill and the various consumer (patient) groups which have developed in the last decade.

Various professionals have predicted that the 1990s will be the decade during which Mental Illness joins physical diseases in the perceptions of the public, the mental health system, and the primary consumers of mental illness and their loved ones. Let's hope so.

Donald R. Self

REFERENCES

Frank, G.F. and M.S. Kamlet (1985). Direct Costs and Expenditures for Mental Health Care in the United States in 1980. *Hospital and Community Psychiatry,* 36.

Presidents Commission on Mental Health (1978). *Report to the President – 1978,* Vol. I-IV. Washington: Governmental Printing Office.

Self, Donald R. (1989). *Alcoholism Treatment Marketing: Beyond T.V. Ads and Speeches.* New York: The Haworth Press, Inc.

Self, Donald R. and James W. Busbin (1990). *Marketing for Health and Wellness Programs.* New York: The Haworth Press, Inc.

Introduction

Donald R. Self

The public mental health (PMH) system is, in many ways, an excellent example of the differences between marketing in a for-profit context and service delivery by a human service agency. The services of the system are considered as "unsought" services by many primary consumers (clients). Practitioners contend with multiple publics of interest including regulators on a local, state, and national level; secondary consumers (family members and advocacy groups); governing boards; a general public with a high level of stigmatic perceptions (negative demand) of the mentally ill (MI) population.

Determining of objectives (the "bottom line") is difficult because of the lack of precision in instruments designed to measure levels and types of mental illness, as well as substantially different objectives among the various publics of interest. The pricing element of the marketing mix is enigmatic because of the decreased level of governmental funding during recent years and restrictions on targeting for-profit funding sources. Additionally, many of the professionals who exert internal influence on marketing activities have not evolved to an "exchange relationship" basis with either primary or secondary consumers.

Traditionally, sanitariums were "holding tanks" for "crazy" or demented individuals. The development of psychotherapy in the twentieth century evolved the discipline into a "professional-client" relationship approximating the "sales" stage of marketing evolution.

During the 1960s, the distribution system for PMH was both broadened and extended into communities by the Community Mental Health Centers (CMHC). During the 1970s and 1980s, successive cutbacks in funding for mental health through the evolution of the "block grant" process has created somewhat of a hybrid with State programs devoting increased attention to the most chronic and acute cases among lower income groups. The quasi-independent CMHCs are developing multiple funding sources in addition to governmental funds. With the passage of PL-99-660 by the federal government in 1986, community input, including that of primary consumers, has radically altered the decision making process of mental health center management. For the first time, PMH systems are being forced to adopt and adapt many of the principles of the marketing process. An additional element in this evolution is the development of associations of practitioners (such as the National Association of Mental Health Information Officers) and consumer and advocacy groups (such as the National Alliance for the Mentally Ill).

This volume is an admittedly eclectic compilation of current knowledge in PMH marketing, including original research manuscripts, tutorials, and case studies. The task of "adapting" marketing knowledge to the MH field is accomplished with the lead article, written several years ago by Bill Winston, Senior Marketing Editor for The Haworth Press, Inc. and consultant within the industry. Several "market segments" (publics) oriented sections focus on the general public as a target market; primary and secondary consumers as a target market; Referral and Secondary; and the use of marketing tools such as research, promotion, and evaluation.

Basic Marketing Principles for Mental Health Professionals

William J. Winston

INTRODUCTION

Health care marketing has become an important management tool for health administrators during recent years. It has only been an accepted scope of study in research during the last decade. However, marketing has been used in health care for centuries. This is documented in the cases of public health campaigns during the 17th and 18th centuries. It has also been extensively utilized by pharmaceutical firms, hospital supply firms, health maintenance organizations, and public health agencies during the last forty years.

The recognition and acceptance of marketing in health care during the 1980s is similar to the rise in importance of finance during the 1970s. Finance was considered the "savior" during this decade as budgeting and financial forecasting became popular in health organizations. Budget directors and controllers were promoted to vice-presidency positions. In comparison, marketing has become the name of the game for the 1980s. Directors of public relations are being promoted to vice-presidents of marketing and planning. Unfortunately, marketing is perceived by many administrators and providers as the future savior. As it will be discussed later, no management tool by itself is a savior.

The development of health care marketing is entering its second phase. During the first half of the 1980s, most of the attention was

This article is reprinted from *Journal of Marketing for Mental Health*, Vol. 1(1) Fall/Winter 1986, pp. 9-20, © The Haworth Press, Inc.

placed on answering the key questions, "what is marketing?" and "why do we need to market?" The second phase during the middle and second half of the 1980s is addressing tools, applications, and sophisticated methodologies for practical use by health administrators and providers.

WHAT IS HEALTH CARE MARKETING?

HEALTH MARKETING is an organized discipline for understanding: (1) how a health marketplace works; (2) the role in which the mental health organization can render optimum services to the marketplace; (3) mechanisms for adjusting production capabilities for meeting consumer demand; and (4) how the mental health organization can assure patient satisfaction.

COMPONENTS OF HEALTH CARE MARKETING

Marketing includes a variety of functions, such as:

1. MARKETING RESEARCH which describes the collection of information about an organization's internal and external environment;
2. MARKETING PLANNING which is the framework for identifying, collecting, and capturing select segments in the marketplace;
3. MARKETING STRATEGY DEVELOPMENT which relates to new service development and actions to be taken for taking advantage of opportunities and gaps in the marketplace;
4. PUBLIC RELATIONS that describes the action of communicating with the publics that interact with the health organization;
5. FUND DEVELOPMENT which is the solicitation of resources for the organization or special services;
6. COMMUNITY RELATIONS which act as a liaison with the publics served;
7. PATIENT LIAISON who acts as intermediator between the provision of care and the patient;
8. RECRUITMENT for medical providers or staff;

9. INTERNAL MARKETING which includes staff development in marketing, marketing role expectation, and triage efficiency; and
10. CONTRACTING for new modes of delivery, such as preferred provider organizations, IPAs, or HMOs.

MARKETING AS A SUBSYSTEM OF MANAGEMENT

Marketing is one function of management. It is integrated with other management subsystems of PRODUCTION, FINANCE, and HUMAN RESOURCES. MARKETING determines the needs of the consumer in the marketplace and lays out a plan for satisfying these needs. Production, finance, and human resources follow this lead and initiate the process of satisfying consumer needs through service provision.

TYPES OF HEALTH MARKETING

There are many applications of marketing in mental health. Some of these applications include marketing for: services, patients, new staff, donors, social causes, creative ideas, goodwill, staff morale, public relations, provider relations, community relations, political and lobbyist activities, new products, fund raising, patient relations, contracting, mergers, joint venturing and acquisitions.

BASIC PREMISES OF HEALTH CARE MARKETING

Before implementing a marketing program, some basic premises must be established about marketing. These include:

1. The patient is a client. There is an exchange process occurring between the consumer and supplier. Even with extensive insurance coverage, every client exchanges time, money, discomfort, and anxiety in obtaining a health service.
2. The best outcome of marketing is a patient or client referral.
3. All providers must continue to assess the effectiveness of their services and not be satisfied to assume they are good just because people use them.

4. Like a new suit of clothes, services must pass initial examination by clients and continue to hold up after the time of initial purchase by the consumer.
5. Marketing is a management tool. It does not offer all the answers to effectively operating a successful organization. It must be blended among financial management, human resource management, strategic planning, and economic analysis.

TEN KEY QUESTIONS ANSWERED BY MARKETING

Marketing supplies answers to the following basic questions for the mental health service:

1. What business are we in and what is the purpose for the organization's existence?
2. Who is our client?
3. What does our client need?
4. Which markets should the organization be addressing?
5. What are the strengths of the organization?
6. What are the weaknesses of the organization that need to be attended to?
7. Who are our competitors?
8. Which groups (segments/targets) do we want to serve in the community?
9. What are our marketing strategies to communicate to these groups?
10. What strategies should we develop related to pricing, promotion, access, and the types of services offered?

TRADITIONAL VERSUS NEWER MARKETING CONCEPTS

The traditional method for understanding marketing is demonstrated by the following relationship:

PRODUCT + SELLING AND PROMOTION = PROFITS THROUGH SALES VOLUME

This relationship is based on the traditional "Madison Avenue" aspect of selling being the most important part of marketing. Selling is only one function of marketing and the real outcome of marketing will be client satisfaction. This is exemplified in the following relationship:

UNDERSTANDING CLIENT NEEDS +
INTEGRATED MARKETING = PROFITS
THROUGH CLIENT SATISFACTION

Integrated marketing includes RESEARCHING THE ENVIRONMENT, DEVELOPING A MARKETING PLAN, and CREATING COMMUNICATION STRATEGIES BASED ON THE RESEARCH AND PLANNING.

Marketing programs which have failed are partly due to a lack of preliminary research, analysis, and planning before implementing communication strategies.

The SELLING CONCEPT focuses on the services; is solely dependent on public relations; and increases revenues through volume. The MARKETING CONCEPT focuses on consumer needs; uses integrated marketing, and increases revenues through consumer satisfaction.

The marketing concept refers to the study or practice of marketing strategies designed to assess consumer preferences about existing or proposed services, implies a direction to deliver services which meet these preferences and needs, and establishes a criterion of effectiveness so that consumers' health needs are satisfied by the services.

PUBLICS, MARKET, EXCHANGE PROCESS

Every organization conducts its business in an environment of both internal and external PUBLICS. A public is a distinct group of people or organizations that have an actual or potential interest or impact on the mental health organization. For example, publics for a psychiatric hospital would be the media, government agencies, other health organizations, the population in the community, medical providers, and its employees.

A mental health organization functions through the exchange process in a MARKET. A market is a process where a minimum of two groups possess resources they want to exchange for some benefit. It is the matching of demand and supply.

Every marketplace has an EXCHANGE. Exchange involves mutual satisfaction of the groups involved. There must be two parties and each must have something that is valued by the other party. For example, patients exchange time, money, discomfort, anxiety, and inconvenience for the services provided.

THE MARKETING MIX

Just as everyone who has studied economics remembers the basic principles of demand and supply, a marketer always is able to fall back on the foundation of the MARKETING MIX. The marketing mix is the mixture or blending of select characteristics of the organization that are utilized to achieve some marketing objective and communicate with a select public.

There are five components of the marketing mix:

1. *PRICING:* This is becoming an important area of health marketing. It can include the direct costs, indirect costs, opportunity costs, discounting, prepayment plans, contracting, co-payments, credit terms, and deductibles. All organizations must price their services to be able to earn a normal profit which is the amount necessary to keep operations and some capital investment going. Normal profits are a regular part of operating costs. Some factors which must be included in the pricing of a service include: demand characteristics for the service, pricing by competitors, consumer expectations for pricing, possible effects on other services provided by the organization, legal aspects, competitive reaction to changes in prices, profitability, and the psychology of the consumer. Some pricing strategies include COMPETITIVE PRICING which sets the price at the "going rate" in the marketplace; MARKET PENETRATION which sets a below-competition price to capture additional market share; SKIMMING which is useful in launching a new service for which the initial price might sustain a high price; and VARIABLE PRICING based on seasonal fluctuations.

2. *PRODUCT:* Marketing strategies can be developed related to the physical characteristics of the products and services provided.

These characteristics include: quality of care, atmospherics, style, size, brand name, service, warranties, types of medical providers, quality of staff interactions, level of technology, and research activities. A mental health organization must have an attractive service which offers some value to the consumer. These values have to satisfy the needs of the consumer. Every new service needs to be researched, have the market screened for potential acceptance, tested for performance levels, and finally, launched into the market selectively. Typically, mental health organizations offer an array of different services. Therefore, a PRODUCT PORTFOLIO needs to be established which plans out the kind of PRODUCT/SERVICE MIX most readily acceptable for the market served.

3. *PLACE:* A key aspect of developing marketing strategies is related to access to the service. The place component of the marketing mix consists of the characteristics of service distribution, modes of delivery, location, transportation, availability, hours and days opened, appointments, parking, waiting time, and other access considerations. Some strategies have included opening a health center on weekends or in the evenings, hiring security guards for evenings, lighting parking lots, possessing excellent triage systems for small amounts of waiting time locating near public transportation, and changing the mode of delivery to include home services.

4. *PROMOTION:* The promotional strategies relate to methods for communicating to the publics. Promotion can include advertising, public relations, personal selling, sales promotion, and publicity. A PROMOTIONAL MIX needs to be established by blending advertising, sales promotion, personal selling, health education, and publicity. The three main ingredients of external communication are the provision of INFORMATION about the service, PERSUASION, and INFLUENCE to use the service if needed. When using promotional strategies, the basic factors to consider are: the availability of funds, the stage of the life cycle the service is in (see next section), the nature of the service, the nature of the market, and the intensity of the competition.

5. *PEOPLE:* All staff, medical providers board members and volunteers are "marketing representatives" of the mental health organization. Human interaction between staff and clients form the client's perception of the service more than any other attribute.

SERVICE/PRODUCT LIFE CYCLE

Just as the human life cycle, every product or service experiences its own unique life cycle. This life cycle includes phases of INTRODUCTION, GROWTH, MATURITY, and DECLINE.

Introduction Phase: In this phase the service is planned for, researched, and developed. It is then introduced into the marketplace for the first time. During this phase, it is usual to experience a considerable amount of technical innovation, research and development, experimentation, initial production and delivery problems, the determination of modes of delivery and channels for distribution, and the development and emergence of the initial marketing mix and promotional strategies. Most strategies relate to informing the publics about the service, educating them about their cost-effectiveness, and instructing them on how to use and obtain the service.

Growth Phase: Expansion occurs and the service becomes accepted by the community. Increased utilization materializes and more resources are inputted into the production process. Typically, new channels for distribution and delivery are created, competitors start to enter the marketplace, attempts are made to entrench the new service in the market by brand loyalty, and emphasis is placed on developing a strong referral network by concentrating on consumer satisfaction.

Maturity Phase: Most mental health organizations are in the maturity phase. This is usually the longest phase for the organization. The market becomes oversaturated with many similar services and competitors. Utilization and revenues tend to level off. Innovation is attempted by modifying the original service to attract new publics or segments, the development of new services begins, and promotion tends to emphasize the reputation of the organization, its history, quality of service, and reliability and integrity.

Decline: Most organizations will not experience a major decline phase which ends in the termination of the organization or service. Utilization and revenues usually decline in this phase dramatically, competition becomes aggressive, many new services are attempted for salvation of the organization, and planned obsolescence is a possibility for the original service. Of course, many products and services have indeterminate life cycles while others are very transitory due to trends. No sooner is one service started than another must be in the design stage to eventually replace or complement it.

THE MARKETING PLANNING PROCESS

A key tool in marketing is the development of a formal written MARKETING PLAN. Unfortunately, most mental health organizations jump the gun and concentrate on implementing strategies and tactics before a solid foundation is established through planning. Many marketing failures occur due to the omission of the planning process. A marketing plan is a framework which lays out the specific steps to market the health service. Marketing planning allows the organizations to: evaluate the marketplace, identify strengths and weaknesses, identify segments to market to, penetrate the market, capture a select market share, and achieve a key positioning/ image within the community.

There are four main components of marketing: ORGANIZA- TION, RESEARCH, CREATIVITY PHASE, and CONTROL.

The ORGANIZATIONAL PHASE of the marketing planning process begins by setting up a marketing committee within the organization. This committee should minimally include the director of marketing, executive director, director of patient services, and a representative from the board. It is important to obtain organizational support for the function of marketing. The committee can be helpful in developing relationships and support from providers, board members, and the staff. A marketing philosophy has to be established by the organization for effectiveness. The MARKET- ING MISSION should be established. It will answer "What business are we in?", "What is the purpose for our existence?", and "Why are we marketing and what main markets are we addressing?" The mission lays a framework for developing the entire marketing program. Then MARKETING GOALS AND OBJECTIVES give us some guidelines for developing the specifics of the program. Marketing goals will outline broad desired results or outcomes we hope to achieve through marketing. The objectives will define the goals by describing specific, measurable outcomes that are to be achieved. For example, a goal could be a broad statement related to increasing utilization. The objective would specify a certain percentage of increased utilization within a time constraint.

The second phase of marketing is the MARKETING RESEARCH OR AUDITING area. Marketing research provides key internal and external information as background to identify trends in the marketplace and help in creating cost effective strategies. The audit should include the collection of information related to: DEMOGRAPHIC FACTORS (i.e., age, sexual mix of the population, region, county size, population growth, climate, etc.); ECONOMIC FACTORS (i.e., income, occupations, industry trends, etc.); PSYCHO-GRAPHIC FACTORS (i.e., lifestyle, values, interests, personality traits, etc.); INDUSTRIAL FACTORS (i.e., competition, health system trends, legislation, lobbyist activities, new modes of delivery, reimbursement trends, etc.); and INTERNAL FACTORS (i.e., quantity and quality of staff, training needs, staff knowledge of marketing and their role in marketing the organization, etc.). After the collection of background information is completed, an OPPOR-TUNITY/RISK ANALYSIS is done. This activity identifies trends from the audit that possibly relate to potential new services and gaps in the marketplace that our organization could fill. The analysis also examines risks to avoid. The outcome of this phase is the identification of market TARGETS that will be marketed to by our programs. First the audit should allow the administrator to subdivide the marketplace into distinct segments which might merit an individual marketing program. After the development of this laundry list of segments, a more finite list of primary and secondary targets can be made. It is not feasible to market every segment. Therefore, the marketing strategies are directed toward select market targets in the marketplace. The primary and secondary targets will consist of those publics in the market which the organization can serve effectively and offer the greatest opportunities.

The three main types of segmentation and targeting are UNDIF-FERENTIATED, DIFFERENTIATED, and CONCENTRATED. Undifferentiated targeting relates to mass marketing whereby it is hoped that the right targets will be communicated by the marketing to everyone. Since finances are limited throughout health care it is important to differentiate your marketing activities. Differentiated targeting identifies a few key targets to address. Concentrated targeting limits the targets to one or two select groups. It has been proven to be cost-effective to approach targeting from a differentiated or concentrated approach rather than from an undifferentiated approach.

It is important to remember that understanding your target's, or consumer's behavior is the backbone of the marketing process. Mental health professionals have an advantage in clinical training in behavior which can be used to analyze consumer behavior.

The CREATIVE PHASE of the planning process includes the development of STRATEGIES AND TACTICS. Strategies and tactics are the specific actions which will be taken to communicate to select target groups with the satisfaction of specific goals and objectives in mind. The first step for strategy development is to develop POSITIONING STRATEGIES. Positioning provides an understanding of how people perceive the organization and identifies how the organization is unique in the marketplace. The underlying philosophy of marketing is to position the organization in the minds of the consumers. Positioning can be related to the quality of the staff, the location, pricing of services, access, and other characteristics of the organization that are unique. The marketing strategies and tactics can be developed by itemizing actions that are directed at marketing a select service. An example of a strategy would be the decision to advertise to a select target group. The tactic would then describe the type of ad, location, size, and color. Strategies can be developed according to the five Ps of the marketing mix discussed earlier: PRICE, PLACE, PRODUCT, PROMOTION or PEOPLE. They can also be developed according to the phase of the life cycle in which the organization fits.

The CONTROL PHASE of the marketing process includes developing a MARKETING BUDGET, IMPLEMENTATION TIME LINE, ORGANIZATIONAL CHART FOR MARKETING, and a CONTROL SYSTEM to monitor the plan's effectiveness. The budget forecasts all of the direct and indirect expenses for developing, implementing, and controlling the marketing plan. The time line outlines specific dates and times for the planning, strategy implementation, and control phases. The organizational chart describes the lines of authority and reporting requirements for the marketing function. The directors of marketing should definitely have planning, public relations, and fund development reporting to them. Direct access to the executive director and a representative of the board may prevent future implementation problems. The control system outlines when and how the marketing program will be monitored for effectiveness. The control system measures the performance of the marketing program against the expected outcomes, or in this case, the goals and objectives that were established in the first phase of the marketing plan. It provides a guideline for pinpointing any problems or deviations and a mechanism for adjusting the plan if necessary, and it accumulates data for future marketing planning.

Marketing plans are essential for successful marketing programs. However, planning does not assure success but it does provide a disciplined approach to marketing and can minimize risks. The marketing plan specifies by service who will do what, when, where, and how, to accomplish the marketing goals and objectives in the most efficient manner. The plan identifies opportunities, coordinates efforts to attract new clients, stimulates creativity in the organization, supports innovation, and allocates resources more effectively. There is an old saying that a marketer needs to "plan the work and work the plan." This means that a lot of planning is useless unless it is implemented carefully. Implementation is as important as developing a plan. The plan is a guideline. It can be changed and adjusted over a long time frame. This is important because marketing is also a long-term process. Results do not occur overnight. Unrealistic expectations about marketing being a miracle worker are one of the major causes of failure. Marketing can be a major management resource for the mental health organization if it is understood and applied effectively through the planning process.

The role of marketing in health care organizations has never been more important. This is reflective of the most competitive mental health care marketplace in history. Mental health organizations are examining new and entrepreneurial ways in which to deliver their services in response to this changing marketplace.

Chronic Mental Illness: Marketing a Wellness Approach at the State and Local Level

Richard E. Plank
Duncan G. LaBay

SUMMARY. Research sponsored by the Robert Wood Johnson Foundation has reaffirmed the presence of the so-called "NIMBY" or not-in-my-backyard attitude toward the placement of a variety of public facilities including those concerned with the maintenance and improvement of mental health. This finding is indicative of the general larger problem of the stigma of mental illness. This paper examines these problems and suggests that nonprofit and governmental policy makers and providers adopt a strategic and tactical marketing perspective for dealing with the issue. Based on the problem and current environment a wellness perspective is suggested as a long term strategy that makes sense and appears workable.

Richard E. Plank, PhD, is Assistant Professor of Marketing at The University of Lowell. Address correspondence to the author at The University of Lowell, Falmouth Hall 205 I, Lowell, MA 01854. Duncan G. LaBay, PhD, is Assistant Professor of Marketing at The University of Lowell. Address correspondence to the author at The University of Lowell, Falmouth Hall 205 G, Lowell, MA 01854.

INTRODUCTION

Mental illness and the health care associated with it continues to be a major and troublesome issue in all parts of our society. As Caldwell (1990) notes, chemical dependency and mental health services continue to be the most problematic employer-provided benefits in terms of cost and utilization control. Frank and McGuire (1990) discuss current legislative initiatives and their impact on federal, state, and local governmental roles and responsibilities. Scallet (1990), Lave and Goldman (1990), and Taube, Goldman, and Salkever (1990) all address the problems of financing with specific reference to the role of Medicare and Medicaid.

George-Perry (1988) has noted that mental health costs are rising at more than 15% per year and now comprise about 25% of all health care expenditures. Demand for such services is directly related to insurance coverage, with one study suggesting that those without insurance would spend about 25% as much as those with coverage (McGlynn et al., 1988). Criticism is also evident as Savitz (1990) has suggested that inpatient psychiatric facilities are the most overused of health care benefits, and that some hospitals are creating rather than responding to real needs. Caldwell (1990) notes a number of insurance company representatives who make similar indictments.

One of the major problems facing mental health practitioners is what appears to be an overwhelming negative image that is associated with their work (Nelson and Barbaro, 1985). Three recent studies, one done in the state of Missouri (1989), one from South Carolina (Craft, 1990), and a national study sponsored by the Robert Wood Johnson Foundation program on mental illness (April, 1990), illustrate the current perspectives of the population on mental health. One other related study of interest has also been reported in the academic literature, a segmentation study by Stone, Warren, and Stevens (1990).

The Missouri study, consisting of 1012 responses to a telephone survey, is promising in that residents of that state appear to be fairly knowledgeable and tolerant of people with mental health disorders. However, about 20% of the respondents thought a larger percentage of mentally ill people are dangerous than is the case; some 48%

overestimated the unpredictability of the mentally ill; and almost half thought mental retardation is a mental illness.

The South Carolina study (Craft, 1990) surveyed 500 state residents by telephone. Some 72% of the respondents felt there is still a considerable stigma attached to mental illness. With regard to possible recovery, 62% felt people with mental illness could recover; 29% were neutral; and 7% felt that these people could not recover. The South Carolina poll was commissioned to compare its residents' attitudes to national statistics. In general, South Carolina residents appear more knowledgeable than the nation as a whole, but also perceive a greater stigma attached to those with mental illness.

Stone, Warren, and Stevens (1990) reported an attempt to segment the mental health services market from the perspective of the importance of different mental health services. Using a telephone survey method, the research obtained information from 387 respondents located in a western city of 350,000. Respondents rated 13 programs on a 5 point importance scale. Services included programs for stress, child/teen behavior disorders, depression, substance abuse, child abuse, and eight other programs. A cluster analysis of the data fit six segments which differed on demographics including sex, family income, occupation of respondent, and the presence of children under 18 living at home. Some 72.4% of the sample were female. Of the six segments, the largest, 28.4%, felt that none of the services were important. The second and third largest groups were the concerned, who thought all the services were important, and the abusive behavior group, who thought teen depression and suicide and substance abuse were important programs. The authors argue that the study demonstrates unique segments, and that the importance of services is a useful way to describe the market for targeting. Since the authors measured nothing in common with the other studies quoted above, it is difficult to relate them.

Unpublished research funded by the Robert Wood Johnson Foundation Program on Chronic Mental Illness (RWJ) has documented national public attitudes toward chronic mental illness (April 1990). In this two-tiered study, a series of depth interviews with national opinion leaders and focus groups with residents of various American cities were conducted. The results of this qualitative research were used to develop a national survey, conducted by telephone with 1326 adults from a national sampling frame. The findings of this study will be examined in detail, in order to better understand how to strategically and tactically deal with the various problems associated with the provision of mental health services.

ROBERT WOOD JOHNSON FOUNDATION STUDY

Opinion Leaders' Responses

The opinion leaders were nationally known people with interest and expertise in mental health. Eighteen people were contacted with a 93% response rate. This group provided a number of useful comments and observations about mental health and the general public, which was used to help shape the telephone survey instrument. In addition, their responses and suggestions are valuable in understanding how to deal with the various problems at a practical level:

1. A major problem is the public's view that people who suffer from mental health problems commit violent acts. In addition, the public wants to stay away from people who are "not like me" and therefore put into the category of strange and frightening.
2. While much of this derives from the vestiges of 19th century notions regarding insane asylums, the news media are considered guilty of perpetuating these beliefs by their treatment of mainly negative stereotyping and portrayal of people with mental illness as violent. Actually only about 1% of mentally ill people are prone to violence, according to experts in the field.
3. The opinion leaders see as a major problem the general public's lack of knowledge about mental illness, although they believe knowledge levels to be slowly improving. A key reason is the emergence of mental health advocacy groups which have brought to the general public better communication about mental illness and the needs of the mentally ill. Yet fear of the mentally ill is still the major problem. Much of the public's known interaction with mentally ill people consists of those who are also homeless, thus causing further negative impressions.

Focus Group Results

Four focus groups were conducted in the Philadelphia area and Columbus, Ohio. The four groups were composed as follows: upscale women, downscale women, upscale men, and downscale men. The existence of the "NIMBY" syndrome was evident in all groups. All groups expressed significant concern over the placement of mainstreaming apartments and homes for mentally ill people. Among male focus groups, particular concerns included the fear of violence and the unknown, concerns about the lack of appropriate supervision, and fears of declining property values.

The focus group participants felt that negative media coverage plays an important role in shaping these attitudes. Interesting, and very troublesome, is the finding that the word "chronic" was usually interpreted to mean "hopeless" or "not treatable," which obviously contributes to negative attitudes toward the mentally ill. Thus these people believe that institutionalization is the best solution for the mentally ill. However, the focus group participants have very little confidence in mental health professionals, especially the government run facilities.

NATIONAL ATTITUDE SURVEY

The national attitude survey was conducted by telephone on a probability sample, including unlisted numbers, and generated 1326 respondents. An average respondent took 29 minutes to complete the interview. Sex and age characteristics were reasonably equivalent to current national statistics, thus suggesting the sample is probably a good representation of the sample frame, at least in terms of demographics. The following key findings emerged:

1. The American public believes that mental illness has increased in the past 20 years and some 89% consider it a serious problem for our society.
2. About 30% report they or someone in their family have sought mental health services at some time in their lives.

3. Americans do not see themselves as very well informed about mental illness and 60% indicate they should know more.
4. Mass media is our society's main source of information, yet 66% of the respondents question to some degree the believability of the information.
5. Americans do believe that anyone can become mentally ill (74%) and that it can be cured (74%), but only 54% believe that keeping a normal life in the community will help a person get better.
6. Sixty-five percent of the respondents believe there is still a lot of stigma attached to mental illness.
7. Over 90% of Americans believe that mental illness can be caused by physical disturbances, environmental conditions such as stress, and by alcoholism or drug abuse.
8. The "Not in My Backyard" (NIMBY) phenomenon appears to be a real problem. Fourteen percent of respondents admitted their neighborhood has opposed some sort of public facility in the past five years and half of those said the opposition was successful.
9. Approximately 20 different types of facilities were rated by respondents and fell into three groups. The most acceptable for most people were schools, day care centers and medical clinics. In the middle were group homes for mentally retarded, homeless shelters, and drug and alcohol treatment centers. Absolutely not acceptable to most people were group homes for AIDS patients, prisons, and commercial or industrial facilities such as shopping malls, factories, and garbage landfills.
10. Of the eight different chronic mental health facilities, most fell in the lower end of the second tier of facilities.
11. Income level was the single best predictor of the acceptability of placing facilities in neighborhoods, with affluent neighborhoods being the most likely to raise opposition to facilities.
12. Using the DYG Environmental Scanning Program it was found that "NIMBYs" are pessimistic about the future, risk averse, competitive, and less tolerant of differences.
13. "NIMBYs" are also less likely to believe that anyone can get mental illness and that these people can get well and return to productive lives.

Summary of Research Findings

The findings are troublesome, but not unexpected. That a stigma exists is well documented, e.g., Nelson and Barbaro (1985). Marmor and Gill (1989) note that the share of GNP devoted to mental health care continues to decline, while the share for physical health care continues to rise. Rochefort (1988) has noted the cyclical nature of mental health system program activity as a way to understand health care policy, but suggests a broader model to help understand policy development. While Rochefort rejects the cyclical model, it is clear that mental health attitudes, in part, stem from incoherent policies on the part of the national, state, and local governments. These incoherent policies are in turn probably driven to some extent by the attitudes of our legislators, which reflect the attitudes of the general public. The RWJ research clearly points out what can be construed as misinformation, lack of knowledge, and social bias. These are major contributors to the lack of acceptance of public mental health initiatives, and hinder the development of cogent policies at all levels to deal with what is obviously a pressing problem.

The single study by Stone, Warren, and Stevens (1990) is interesting, but has limited value to policy makers. It has a primarily female response base and is done in one city using a telephone survey technique. It asked respondents what was important to them, but did not assess their knowledge of the services in question or how to deliver them. Replication with a more representative sample and integrating other issues of importance will give policy makers guidance in developing strategy.

DEVELOPING COGENT
MENTAL HEALTH CARE POLICIES
AT THE STATE AND LOCAL LEVEL

It is clear from the RWJ research and other sources that in order to develop effective mental health care policies, several related problems must be overcome:

1. The American public has a very negative view toward mental health problems, care givers, and government policies and programs. While there is evidence of improvement, the situation is not conducive to developing easily understood, acceptable, effective, and efficient mental health care programs and policies.
2. The American public has little knowledge about mental health in general. What they do know is often incorrect or at best misleading. Again, while there is some evidence of improvement, further education is obviously necessary.
3. Although not much is known about the views of American governmental representatives, the history of mental health legislation at all levels leads one to believe that legislators have the same attitudes as their constituents and may consider the issue politically difficult.
4. The economy is in difficult times at both the national level and in many states. The current recession and federal budget deficit, coupled with the decline of state tax receipts, make it difficult to develop funding for new initiatives for mental health, or even to fund existing ones.

Taking a strategic long term perspective and understanding how to deal with these problems requires a structured approach to the problem. Utilizing a strategic marketing model allows a holistic view of the problem and provides a framework to ask the relevant questions and develop a cogent program. Some aspects of this have already been discussed by Ambrose and Lennox (1988), but not primarily from a policy-making perspective.

Figure 1 provides an overview of the strategic planning process from the perspective of the Mental Health Policy Maker. Strategic analysis requires that the participant begin the process with an analysis of both the internal and external constraints facing that policy maker. Internal constraints include the issues of developing objectives, understanding the resource limitations, and examining the strengths and weaknesses of the policy making body and significant others who are involved in the process. External analysis requires the examination of the consumers, other publics, competition, and economic conditions to be faced in the short and long term. It also

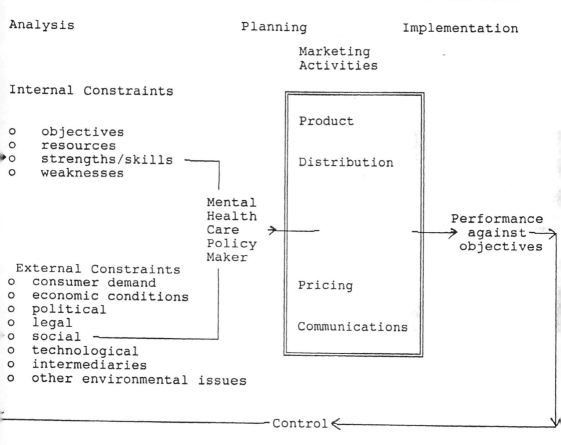

FIGURE 1
STRATEGIC ANALYSIS AND PLANNING FOR MENTAL HEALTH POLICY

Analysis   Planning   Implementation

                                  Marketing
                                  Activities

Internal Constraints

o   objectives   Product
o   resources
o   strengths/skills ───   Distribution
o   weaknesses

                    Mental
                    Health
                    Care   →   → Performance
                    Policy   against ──→
                    Maker   objectives

  External Constraints
o   consumer demand   Pricing
o   economic conditions
o   political
o   legal   Communications
o   social ──
o   technological
o   intermediaries
o   other environmental issues

──────────────────────────────── Control ←─────────────────────────

involves analysis of social conditions affecting policy development, any technology that may play a role, and finally the role of various intermediaries and other publics who may impact on or be impacted by the policies developed. From a marketing perspective the policies developed become the strategic product mix, because they dictate the various programs that will be implemented. Those programs and approaches to improving mental health are in fact the product. Distribution issues concern who will deliver the various mental health services. Communications refers to the broad problem of communicating to the various publics the policies and offerings that are the result of the product and distribution decisions. While this is an important decision, it is clearly not the only decision. Programs that only consider communication issues will not be effective. Price concerns not only how programs will be priced, but who will pay for the services and how they will pay for them.

The following discussion will outline in some detail the issues that must be dealt with in developing and implementing policies. While the focus will be at the state level of activity, the same process is useful for local agencies. Each of the major areas of Figure 1 will be discussed in some detail. A specific strategic thrust, that of developing a mental wellness approach, will be discussed as a method of generating mental health policies. The concept of wellness is one which has been developing over the past 10 years, mostly in the area of physical health. Its extension to the mental health area seems most appropriate.

THE WELLNESS CONCEPT

State and local mental health professionals have a number of strategic directions from which to choose. One option is, of course, to do nothing and to continue on the current path. There are a number of other options available such as focusing on legislation to better enforce existing civil rights, or to provide completely new and different programs. A movement that is gaining force in the general medical profession in this country is the idea of wellness (Busbin, 1990a). The wellness philosophy suggests that health care consumers not only take a more active role in their health care (Reeder,

1972), but that the focus of health care be preventative (Bloch, 1984).

Wellness as a philosophy has been enthusiastically endorsed by business firms which recognize that healthy employees are productive employees (Moretz, 1988; Kitrell 1988). While wellness activities primarily cover physical well being, Welter (1988) and others have noted that stress management is often included in wellness programs.

The literature on wellness is beginning to develop and has been reviewed by Busbin (1990b). Among the shortages in the literature is the problem of policy leadership, both by the federal government as well as the insurance industry. In addition, little work has been done in the area of consumer psychology as it relates to wellness. An exception is the work of Plank and Gould (1990) who find that wellness-type activities are related to the health consciousness of individuals as well as to their predisposition for a scientific orientation to health care.

Recent unpublished work by Plank and Gould (1991) indicates how difficult it is to reach health conscious people. The research examined middle-class adults in two northeastern markets. It assessed the relationship of health consciousness (which correlates highly to wellness-type activities) to media habits and demographics. In both samples, numbering 495 adults total, neither demographics nor media habits were significant predictors of wellness and health consciousness. About all that could be said is that health conscious consumers seem to watch and listen to more health programs.

Much descriptive and prescriptive work has been done on dental wellness (Budden and Browning, 1990), marketing to older adults (Self and Wilkinson, 1990), adolescents (Self and Self, 1990), and implementation of wellness programs in a resource-constrained public institution (Fugate, 1990). In addition, both Blades (1990) and Bart (1990) have assessed the marketing of wellness by hospitals.

The wellness phenomenon continues to develop and snowball into the philosophy of choice for health care consumption in this country. The idea of prevention, long the predominant philosophy in dental care, is becoming more dominant in physical care in general. With greater numbers of educated people taking control over their own health care decision process, the wellness approach as a philosophy becomes more appropriate. There are a number of compelling arguments for this kind of approach, both social and economic. Clearly, healthy citizens are more productive citizens. If prevention results in less illness and thus less cost of total care, resources from health care can be diverted to other pressing areas for the benefit of society. This growth and development of wellness has occurred despite the lack of well defined programs on the part of federal, state and local governments and the insurance industry. It has primarily been driven by the business community, which assumes a positive relationship between healthy employees and productivity and thus competitiveness.

INTERNAL CONSTRAINTS

Internal constraints such as resources are likely to vary from state to state and between local agencies within a given state. In general, the mood of the public seems to be less supportive of government spending at all levels. Economic difficulties currently exist in the majority of states. A major and continuing problem facing most states and local agencies is the lack of cogent and consistent policies on the part of the federal government. While it is arguably true that mental health programs are best delivered on a state and local level, there exists a need for the federal government to provide guidelines and incentives, if not outright funding, to allow local units to develop long term approaches to mental health care.

EXTERNAL CONSTRAINTS

Recent research, as noted above, paints a clear if not exactly supportive picture of the public position towards mental health programs. The following summarizes the various research findings and addresses the current economic situation.

1. The public is not very knowledgeable about mental illness and for the most part does not even differentiate mental illness from mental disabilities. In addition, many believe a large proportion of people who have chronic mental illness are dangerous to the public, when in fact the true figure is estimated to be 1%.
2. This lack of knowledge translates to the belief that programs to de-institutionalize the mentally ill, by placing them in regular living arrangements, are wrong. The result is public resistance to these kinds of arrangements in their neighborhoods.
3. There is little in the way of consistent federal, and hence state and local, programs with regards to mental illness. Some states appear more active than others; some localities do more; but there is no consistent national policy.
4. While the media have done a better job of portraying mental illness, there is much room for improvement.
5. In general, the public has poor attitudes toward mental health professionals and is concerned with misdiagnosis. A significant portion of the population still does not believe mental illness can be cured. In addition, the existence of a large homeless population and attitudes toward them by many citizens further exacerbates these problems.
6. This all points to a general stigma about mental illness which is well documented and is "real."
7. The general economic climate is such that it is difficult to procure large amounts of extra funding, regardless of how meritorious, since excess funds do not exist. The recession coupled with the federal budget deficit makes it difficult at that level. Many states are struggling with deficits of their own in 1991.

DEVELOPING A POLICY

Given the brief sketch of the internal and external environment as faced by state and local mental health policy makers, how do they go about formulating a long-term strategy to improve the mental health of society? As suggested above, a long-term solution to our mental health problems may be best approached by following a wellness perspective. The key to such a program is the development at the state level, with federal support, of a series of programs or products that deal with the prevention as well as the cure of mental illness. The distribution of these programs, or who will carry them out, the promotion of these programs, and the pricing of these programs are all critical if the entire perspective is to be successful.

Product

The product is a series of programs aimed at the mental health problem. This will include the usual programs aimed at cure, but will also include a number of efforts to incorporate the notion of wellness into the mental health arena. Education programs at all levels must be developed. Grade school, high school, college, and general public awareness programs must be developed noting that mental health problems are both preventable and curable. Specific efforts modeled after the stress management programs currently incorporated in wellness programs must be initiated to deal with such issues as depression and other preventable mental health problems. Emphasis on curative programs such as neighborhood housing needs to be framed as part of the wellness program. People in wellness programs need to interact with residents of these types of facilities.

Distribution

Distribution is concerned with who will deliver the various programs and how. Distribution is going to be complex. As Busbin (1990b) notes there are six different major parties involved in the wellness movement. Hospitals are major providers of programs. Companies, both profit and nonprofit, provide employee fringe benefit plans that include wellness programs. Insurance companies are the financial foundation on which health care systems in this country are based. There are a number of specialty wellness programs including some related to mental health, such as private addiction clinics. The federal government is the primary policy maker. Finally, employees themselves, or more broadly health care consumers, are part of the program along with any unions which may represent those employees.

Some programs will continue to be delivered by the state. Private enterprise may be appropriate for some of these programs. As noted above, certain drug and alcohol rehabilitation programs that are private have had some success. Wellness programs can and must be delivered by the same variety of providers that deliver them today. Businesses can be expected to be the major catalyst for mental health wellness programs, just as they have been for physical health. The insurance industry must be brought in early and must buy into the preventive notion, providing the necessary financial backing and structure that will ensure acceptance of wellness perspectives. Much as in environmental issues, individual states can take the lead and mandate certain types of programs and approaches. California has been notable in its approach to clean air, and in the longer run for its impact on other states and federal government policies.

Promotion

Promotion concerns itself with providing information about products and services to the user and more generally making consumers aware of the mental illness problem. As noted, consumers have misconceptions about certain aspects of mental illness and many are ignorant of the issues. Advertising is only one facet of promotion, and not the most important element for the long term wellness program being suggested here.

Promotion will be achieved by the nature of some of the services themselves; education is the major example. Education must start early and educational programs must revolve around the idea of wellness and prevention. By starting these programs in the grade schools and continuing them through high school, the next generation of adult citizens will develop more positive images of mental health and act as facilitators of attitude change for the older generations. Drug and alcohol education within the wellness format is obviously an important part of this education.

The major promotional key, otherwise, is the business community, and particularly large organizations which have embraced wellness programs. By convincing these organizations to incorporate specific mental health wellness programs one will reach large numbers of consumers. In addition, major efforts must be made with the media. Efforts must be made to portray mental illness in a positive way. Public relations programs must be developed for the various media, including television, radio, newspaper, and magazines. The entertainment media should be especially targeted for both positive and negative feedback concerning their portrayals of mental illness.

The theme that must pervade all promotional efforts, including advertising, is that of wellness. Mental illness can be prevented and cured. Mental illness must be portrayed in a less negative light.

By allowing the business community and insurance companies to be a major catalyst, one will generate a large amount of promotion geared to developing the market. This is far more promotion than could be achieved by the states or mental health agencies attempting direct advertising to the general public. Prior research (Plank and Gould, 1991) has shown that it is difficult to target wellness and other health-oriented advertising using the general media. Thus, indirect promotion is likely to be much more effective in both the short and long run.

Pricing

Pricing refers to not only how much will be paid, but by whom and how. Since third party carriers are so critical in this area, insurance firms must have input into this process. The business community in general is critical. Kitrell (1988) has documented savings for companies that have wellness programs. Such types of savings for mental health programs establish the price/value of the programs.

CONCLUSION

What has been suggested by this paper is that mental health policy makers take a long term market oriented view to developing mental health policy and programs. Given the current general stigma regarding mental illness, and the public's reluctance to support current cures, it has been suggested that a wellness strategy be adopted. While this represents only one possible longer term strategy, wellness provides a positive halo for what most people view as a negative phenomenon. Such a positive halo can change attitudes toward the problem in the long run. The wellness perspective, which suggests that mental illness may be to some extent preventable, makes sense given that physical health activities also are turning more to prevention. Mental health policy makers are obviously in an unenviable position. Short term prospects are negative, both in terms of program funding and attitudes toward mental health. A long term plan needs to be developed.

The wellness phenomenon has been an active movement for nearly a decade. In that time it has worked its way into the consciousness of a large number of consumers and policy makers. A long term approach to mental health under this framework could see similar results in this decade, with perhaps a complete public turnaround in the next 20 to 30 years. A strategic marketing process, concentrating on the development of products, the distribution network, appropriate communications and pricing must be encouraged. Since wellness activities give people a choice framework, such programs are more acceptable to the general public and invite their education. This facilitates education in a positive way and with a positive halo, thus accelerating the process and discouraging opposition. Given the proper programs, the "NIMBY" phenomenon may well become an issue of the past.

BIBLIOGRAPHY

(1989) "Missouri Survey on Mental Illness," *Mental Health Reporter*, (December) Missouri Department of Mental Health.

(1990) "Public Attitudes Toward People with Chronic Mental Illness," Unpublished report prepared by DYG, Inc. for The Robert Wood Johnson Foundation Program on Chronic Mental Illness, (April).

REFERENCES

Ambrose, D.M., and L. Lennox, (1988) "Strategic Market Positions for Mental Health Services," *Journal of Mental Health Administration*, 15 (Spring), 5-9.

Bart, B.D., (1990) "Evaluating the Effectiveness of Wellness Programs: Urban and Rural Hospital Experience," *Health Marketing Quarterly*, 7, 3/4, 219-227.

Blades, H.C., (1990) "Wellness: The Marketing of Health Promotion in America's Heartland Hospitals," *Health Marketing Quarterly*, 7, 3/4, 201-218.

Bloch, P.H., (1984) "The Wellness Movement: Imperatives for Health Care Marketers," *Journal of Health Care Marketing*, 4, 1 (Winter), 9-16.

Budden, M.C., and S.R. Browning, (1990) "The Marketing of Dental Wellness: A Practical Guide for the Practitioner," *Health Marketing Quarterly*, 7, 3/4, 23-32.

Busbin, J.W., (1990a) "Market Evolutions in Health Care and the Emergence of Employee Wellness as a New Product Category," *Health Marketing Quarterly*, 7, 3/4, 7-22.

Busbin, J.W., (1990b) "Surpluses and Shortages in the Study of Wellness Programs: An Assessment of the Field's Development and Call for Academic Research," *Health Marketing Quarterly*, 7, 3/4, 229-249.

Caldwell, B., (1990) "Controversies in Behavioral Health Care," *Employee Benefit Plan Review*, 45, 1 (July), 30,32.

Craft, S., (1990) "South Carolinians Reveal Attitudes Toward Mental Illness," *FOCUS On Mental Health Issues*, 1, 4 (July/August) South Carolina Department of Mental Health, 1-4.

Frank, R.G., and T.G. McGuire, (1990) "Mandating Employer Coverage of Mental Health Care," *Health Affairs*, 9, 1 (Spring), 31-42.

Fugate, D.L., (1990) "Implementing a Wellness Program in a Resource Constrained Public Institution: A Review with Commentary," *Health Marketing Quarterly*, 7, 3/4, 175-188.

George-Perry, S., (1988) "Easing the Costs of Mental Health Benefits," *Personnel Administrator*, 33, 11 (November), 52-57.

Kitrell, A., (1988) "Wellness Plans Can Save Money: Survey," *Business Insurance*, 22, 13 (March 28), 3,10.

Lave, J.R., and H.H. Goldman, (1990) "Medicaid Financing for Mental Health Care," *Health Affairs*, 9, 1 (Spring), 19-30.

Marmor, T.R., and K.C. Gill, (1989) "The Political and Economic Context of Mental Health Care in the United States," *Journal of Health Politics, Policy & Law*, 14, 3 (Fall), 459-475.

McGlynn, E.A., G.S. Norquist, K. Wells, G. Sullivan, and R.P. Liberman, (1988) "Quality-of-Care Research in Mental Health: Responding to the Challenge," *Inquiry*, 25, 1 (Spring), 157-170.

Moretz, S., (1988) "Wellness Programs: Keeping Workers Fit," *Occupational Hazards*, 50, 4 (April), 59-62.

Nelson, G.D., and M. Barbaro, (1985) "Fighting the Stigma: A Unique Approach to Marketing Mental Health," *Health Marketing Quarterly*, 2, 4 (Summer), 89-101.

Plank, R.E., and S.J. Gould, (1990) "Health Consciousness, Scientific Orientation and Wellness: An Examination of the Determinants of Wellness Attitudes and Behaviors," *Health Marketing Quarterly*, 7, 3/4, 65-82.

Plank, R.E., and S.J. Gould, (1991) "Health Consciousness, Media Usage, and Demographics: The Problems with Targeting Promotion to Health Conscious Individuals," Unpublished Working Paper, University of Lowell, Department of Marketing, Lowell, MA.

Reeder, L.G., (1972) "The Patient-Client as a Consumer: Some Observations on the Changing Profession-Client Relationship," *Journal of Health and Social Behavior,* 13, 4 (December), 406-412.

Rochefort, D.A., (1988) "Policymaking Cycles in Mental Health: Critical Examination of a Conceptual Model," *Journal of Health Politics, Policy, & Law,* 13, 1 (Spring), 129-152.

Savitz, A.S., (1990) "Psychiatric Care Overused," *Business Insurance,* 24, 23 (June 4), 29.

Scallet, L.J., (1990) "Paying for Public Mental Health Care: Crucial Questions," *Health Affairs,* 9, 1 (Spring), 117-124.

Self, R.M., and N. Wilkinson, (1990) "Promoting Wellness for Older Adults," *Health Marketing Quarterly,* 7, 3/4, 95-124.

Self, D.R., and R.M. Self, (1990) "The Adolescents: Target Market for Prevention," *Health Marketing Quarterly,* 7, 3/4, 125-139.

Stone, T.R., W.E. Warren, and R.E. Stevens, (1990) "Segmenting the Mental Health Care Market," *Journal of Health Care Marketing*, 10, 1 (March), 65-69.

Taube, C.A., H.H. Goldman, and D. Salkever, (1990) "Medicaid Financing for Mental Health Care," *Health Affairs,* 9, 1 (Spring), 19-30.

Welter, T.R., (1988) "Wellness Programs: Not a Cure-All," *Industry Week,* 236, 4 (February 15), 42-45.

The Relationship of Demographic Characteristics and Importance of Services Offered to Unaided Awareness and Recommendation of Public and Private Mental Health Care Providers

William E. Warren
Robert E. Stevens
Terry R. Stone

SUMMARY. The extent to which demographic characteristics and importance of services offered by mental health providers are related to unaided awareness and recommendation of public and private mental health care providers was assessed. Awareness and recommendation of private providers was found to be stronger among men and among higher income groups. Relative to public providers, these factors were stronger among women and lower income groups. While the services offered do not appear to be strongly related to awareness or recommendation of provider types, some differences were found. Those who are aware of and would recommend a private provider gave higher importance ratings to counseling for suicide and life changes—those who are aware of and would recommend a public provider gave higher ratings to counselling for spouse

William E. Warren, PhD, is Associate Professor of Marketing, Management and Marketing Department at Middle Tennessee State University, MTSU Box 75, Murfreesboro, TN 37132. Robert E. Stevens, PhD, is Professor of Marketing at Northeast Louisiana University. Terry R. Stone is President, Stone and Associates, Boulder, CO.

abuse, depression, and eating disorders, and treatment for major mental illness.

INTRODUCTION

Mental health care is a very large and growing segment of the health care market. Between 1970 and 1986 (the most recent year for which data are available), the total number of mental health services providers increased almost forty-eight percent — from 3005 in 1970 to 4447. However, the dramatic change that has occurred in the "mix" of mental health care providers is even more significant. State and county providers decreased from 310 to 285 or about 8 per cent while private psychiatric hospitals more than doubled, from 150 to 314. VA hospital medical centers providing psychiatric services increased from 115 to 139 (20.9%), and the number of general hospitals with separate psychiatric services increased from 797 to 1351 (69.5%) (Manderscheid and Sonnenschein 1990).

There have also been significant changes in the availability of services provided — inpatient, outpatient, and partial care. Organizations that provided inpatient services increased 75.3% (from 1734 to 3039) however, the total number of inpatient beds decreased almost 50% (from 524,878 to 267,613). As shown in Table 1, most of this decrease can be attributed to the reductions in state and county mental hospitals, but these institutions still accounted for more than forty-four per cent of the total psychiatric beds available for inpatient care (Manderscheid and Sonnenschein 1990).

Table 1

DISTRIBUTION OF INPATIENT BEDS BY TYPE OF PROVIDER

Type Provider	1970 %	1980 %	1986 %
State and County	78.7	57.0	44.5
Private Psychiatric	2.7	6.6	11.3
Non-Federal General Hospitals With Separate Psychiatric Services	4.3	10.7	17.1
VA Medical Centers	9.7	12.3	10.0

Source: Adapted from Manderscheid and Sonnenscheid 1990*

* adds to less than 100% because some miscellaneous types have been omitted

Similarly, the number of outpatient providers increased from 2156 to 2946 (36.6%) but the number of state and county mental hospitals and private psychiatric hospitals that provided outpatient services decreased. The number of organizations providing partial care more than doubled—from 778 to 1943. However, because of redefinition of partial care, these data are not directly comparable (Manderscheid and Sonnenschein 1990).

These changes obviously are profound, particularly so when viewed from a public/private provider perspective—the relative importance of the private sector is increasing at the expense of the public sector. A number of factors may contribute to these changes, such as decreases in federal and state funding, change in public opinion and so forth. However, the growth in private psychiatric hospitals and general hospitals with separate psychiatric services are indicators of the competitiveness of the industry and suggest the need for an organization to develop and implement sound marketing practices in order to compete effectively and efficiently. To do so, an organization must understand its target market and then build a marketing plan that will satisfy that market. However, relatively few mental health services providers appear to have accomplished either of these tasks.

REVIEW OF RELEVANT LITERATURE

Relatively few studies specifically related to the marketing of mental health services have been published and virtually none have addressed the public/private dichotomy. Hoffman and Nelson (1987) have presented the development and implementation of a marketing plan designed for a small child and adolescent inpatient psychiatric unit in a large community hospital. This plan heavily concentrated on the referral network—psychiatrists, pediatricians, school counselors, and clergy. The authors posit that a successful marketing plan must be tied to the goals of the program and its effectiveness evaluated on a fixed schedule. Ambrose and Lennox (1988) have stressed the importance of strategic market positions. In their opinion, as the market environment becomes increasingly competitive, positioning will be the key to success for mental health programs and institutions.

Stone, Warren, and Stevens (1990) reported a study in which six segments of the mental health care market were identified. Further, they concluded "the mental health care market consists of several distinct segments . . . consumers differ on the types of mental health care they are most concerned about and these segments, in turn, have different consumer characteristics" (p.68). However, their study did not address the private/public provider dichotomy.

Mental health services providers can also benefit from the efforts completed in other areas of health care services. Lim and Zallocco (1988) studied determinant attributes in formulation of attitudes toward a variety of health care providers. The dimensions that most clearly differentiated attitudes were personalized care, quality of medical care, and value. In addition, they found that demographic characteristics may influence attitudes.

Other researchers have found that top-of-mind unaided awareness appears to give a competitive edge in building preference among hospitals that are not currently used by consumers (Woodside and Shinn 1988). But, the first hospital that comes to mind is likely to depend on the type of service within hospitals. Consequently, measuring hospital unaided awareness in reference to specific services is likely to be useful.

A variety of approaches to segmentation of various health care markets have been reported. Martin (1988) found that problem analysis is an insightful approach for understanding salient needs among health care consumers. "In a market where notable changes in delivery systems and consumer needs are occurring, this approach provides information that is 'directly' applicable to strategy formulation" (p. 16). Finn and Lamb (1986) examined the relative importance that health care consumers attach to various benefits available in a major metropolitan area hospital as an approach to market segmentation.

Woodside and others (1988) have reported the results of a national segmentation study that extended the work of Finn and Lamb (1986) and Kotler and Clarke (1987). Their study used cluster analysis to classify respondents who preferred hospitals for inpatient care. The groups were based on reasons given for their hospital preferences. Then demographic profiles of the grouped respondents were compared to learn whether several of the groups could be identified efficiently. The study identified four market segments.

PURPOSE OF THE STUDY

Dramatic changes have occurred within the mental health care market over the past several years. Among the most significant changes is the relative decline in importance of public providers and the corresponding increase in private provider importance. However, virtually no research related to the private/public provider dichotomy has been reported.

Previous research has shown that unaided awareness can be key in building preference among hospitals, particularly so when awareness is related to specific health care services. Further, benefits sought has been shown to be a viable basis for mental health care market segmentation. The purpose of the present study was to apply the findings from previous research to an assessment of the public/private dichotomy. More specifically the purposes were to:

1. Assess the extent to which demographic characteristics are related to awareness and recommendation of public/ private providers.
2. Assess the extent to which services offered (or benefits sought) are related to awareness and recommendation of public/private providers.

METHODOLOGY

Data for the study were gathered via telephone. A professional field service group conducted a total of 387 interviews in a western city with a population base of more than 350,000.

Respondents were asked which mental health providers in the area they could name and then which of these providers they would recommend to a friend in need of such services. In addition, respondents were asked to use a scale ranging from most important (1) to least important (5) to rate each of thirteen services/programs that might be offered by a mental health services organization (these are detailed in Tables 4 and 8). Finally, respondents were asked their age, income, and gender.

The providers named by respondents were grouped into public and private and these groups served as the basis for analysis. Both chi square and multiple discriminant analysis (MDA) were utilized as analytic tools.

MDA was employed to determine if the *a priori* defined groups differ with respect to the demographic characteristics and the relative importance of benefits offered by providers. All dimensions were included in the analysis and each had a chance of entering. A step-wise analysis was used requiring a minimum F value of 1.0 to enter. SPSSX Method = Wilks controlled the entry order.

MDA generates linear functions based on the predictor variables that best discriminate among the groups, and it provides an overall test for significant differences among the groups. If a significant difference is determined, the relative importance of each predictor variable in discrimination among the groups is provided, and the dimensions on which the groups differ can be determined. The discriminant function is validated by first estimating the function on half of the sample and then applying the function to the hold-out sample. Because the actual group memberships are known, the percentage of correct classifications can be computed (Frank, Massey, and Morrison 1965).

The canonical loadings (the correlation between the predictor variables and the discriminant function coefficients) are used to minimize the potential "weighting" problems caused by multicollinearity. Futhermore, the loadings can be rotated to aid in interpretation (Perreault, Behrman, and Armstrong 1979). The relative value of the canonical loading for each variable indicates the directional relationship.

Dummy variables were created for each of the demographic characteristics. (For example, if a respondent reported her age as 21, that category was coded 1. Each of the other age categories was then coded 0 for that respondent.) This was done for two reasons. First, virtually all of the demographic characteristics were measured categorically, not continuously — the respondent selected the one age, income, etc. category that described her. Second, this approach provides richer, more descriptive information. For example, instead of merely finding that age is a discriminating variable, the specific age category (i.e., 18-24) that discriminates is shown.

FINDINGS

Overall, unaided awareness of mental health care providers was found to be low. Less than one-third (32%) of the respondents were able to give the name of a provider. Forty-six per cent of the named providers were public and fifty-four per cent were private. Demographic profiles of respondents aware of each provider type are shown in Table 2. Males are more likely to be aware of private providers and awareness of private providers tends to increase as income increases. The opposite is true for those aware of public providers.

The discriminant analysis of demographics produced a discriminant function significant at the .0068 level. The correct classification percentages for the analysis and hold-out portions of the sample

Table 2

DEMOGRAPHIC PROFILE OF MENTAL HEALTH CARE PROVIDERS:
UNAIDED AWARENESS

	Public Providers	Private Providers
Total	57	68
	%	%
Gender		—
Female	86.0	66.2
Male	14.0	33.8
Chi Square 5.4929 1 d.f.		Sig. .0191
Age		
18-24	7.0	7.4
25-34	22.8	26.5
35-44	31.6	32.3
45-54	17.5	17.6
55 and older	21.1	16.2
Chi Square .5794 4 d.f.		Sig. .9653
Income		
Under $10,000	10.5	1.5
$10,000-19,999	24.6	19.1
$20,000-29,999	28.1	22.1
$30,000-39,999	15.8	19.1
$40,000 and over	19.3	25.0
Not reported	1.8	13.2
Chi Square 11.1722 5 d.f.		Sig. .0481

were 66.4 per cent and 62.6 per cent respectively, while the chance proportion is 50 per cent. The differences in the significant discrimination demographic characteristics are presented in Table 3. Purchase intensity group means represent the proportion of a group that is described by a demographic characteristic. For example, 26.47 per cent of those aware of private providers are male. As shown, respondents aware of private providers tend to be male and those aware of public providers tend to have lower income levels.

Generally, respondents aware of each provider type gave similar importance ratings for the services (benefits) that may be offered by a mental health provider. These importance ratings are shown in Table 4. Neither chi square nor t-tests of mean ratings analyses produced significant differences between the two groups. The discriminant analysis produced a discriminant function significant, but at only the .0398 level. The correct classification percentages for the analysis and hold-out groups were 60.8 and 54.6 per cent respectively—the chance proportion is 50 per cent. Those aware of public providers tend to place a somewhat greater degree of importance on counseling for eating disorders, depression, and spouse abuse (see Table 5).

Only about one-fourth of the total respondents could name a mental health provider that they would recommend to a friend in need of such services. However, the majority (78%) of those aware of a mental health provider mentioned one that they would recommend to a friend. The demographic profiles of the type of provider that would be recommended are shown in Table 6. Private pro-

Table 3

DIFFERENCES IN DEMOGRAPHICS: UNAIDED
AWARENESS OF PROVIDER TYPE

	Canonical Loadings	Group Means	
		Public Providers	Private Providers
Demographics			
Male	-1.5697	.2281	.2647
Income <$10,000	3.0279	.1053	.0147
$10,000-19,999	.9428	.2456	.1912
$20,000-29,999	1.0926	.2807	.2206

Wilks' Lambda .8895   Chi "Square 14.163   (4 d. f.)   Sig. .0068

Table 4

UNAIDED AWARENESS OF MENTAL HEALTH CARE PROVIDERS
RELATED TO RELATIVE IMPORTANCE OF BENEFITS

	Public Providers	Private Providers
Total Benefit	Imp. Rat. *	Imp. Rat.*
Counseling for child/ teen beh. prob.	2.51	2.41
Counseling for teen suicide/depress.	2.32	2.41
Counseling for teen substance abuse	2.26	2.40
Counseling for adult substance abuse	2.56	2.72
Counseling for eating disorders	3.39	3.49
Counseling for stress	2.49	2.57
Counseling for anxiety	3.09	3.34
Counseling for depression	2.51	3.03
Counseling for suicide	2.67	2.90
Counseling for life changes	2.82	2.82
Counseling for child abuse	2.47	2.94
Counseling for spouse abuse	2.54	2.65
Treatment for major mental illness	2.71	3.51

* 1 = <u>most</u> important, 5 = <u>least</u> important

Table 5

DIFFERENCES IN IMPORTANCE OF BENEFITS:
UNAIDED AWARENESS OF PROVIDER TYPE

	Canonical Loadings	Group Means	
		Public Providers	Private Providers
Benefits			
Counseling for eating disorders	-.4096	3.3860	3.4411
Counseling for depression	.7006	2.5088	3.0294
Counseling for life changes	-.4193	2.8246	2.8235
Counseling for spouse abuse	.4466	2.5439	3.0882

Wilks' Lambda .9204   Chi Square 10.037 (4 d.f.) Sig. .0398

Note: <u>Lower</u> rating indicates <u>greater</u> importance

Table 6
DEMOGRAPHIC PROFILE OF MENTAL HEALTH CARE PROVIDERS
THAT WOULD BE RECOMMENDED TO FRIEND

	Public Providers	Private Providers
Total	36	62
	%	%
Gender		
Female	88.9	69.4
Male	11.1	30.6
Chi Square 3.31 1 d.f.		Sig. .0509
Age		
18-24	8.3	8.1
25-34	19.4	21.0
35-44	27.8	40.3
45-54	16.7	19.3
55 and older	27.8	11.3
Chi Square 4.69 4 d.f.		Sig. .3206
Income		
Under $10,000	8.3	1.6
$10,000-19,999	33.2	17.7
$20,000-29,999	33.2	25.8
$30,000-39,999	13.9	22.6
$40,000 and over	11.1	24.2
Not reported	.3	8.1
Chi Square 11.10 5 d.f.		Sig. .0488

viders are more likely to be recommended by men and by respondents with higher levels of income – public by women and lower income groups.

The discriminant analysis of demographic characteristics produced a discriminant function significant at the .0056 level. The correct classification percentages for the analysis and hold-out portions of the sample were 68.4 and 65.8 per cent respectively. The differences in the significant discrimination demographic characteristics are shown in Table 7. Those who would recommend a private provider tend to be male while those who would recommend a public provider tend to have lower incomes.

As shown in Table 8, those recommending each type of provider tended to give similar importance ratings for each of the mental health service programs (benefits). Both chi square and t-test of mean ratings failed to produce significant results. The discriminant analysis produced a significant discriminant function, but at only the .0148 level. The correct classification percentages for the analysis and hold-out groups were 75.5 and 68.9 per cent respectively – chance proportion is 50 per cent. Those who would recommend a

Table 7

DIFFERENCES IN DEMOGRAPHICS BETWEEN RECOMMENDED
PROVIDER TYPE

Demographics	Canonical Loadings	Group Means Public Providers	Private Providers
Male	−1.4400	.1111	.3065
Age 18-25	−1.4548	.0833	.0807
Income <$10,000	3.7024	.0833	.0161
$10,000-19,999	1.7821	.3333	.1774
$20,000-29,999	1.2848	.3333	.4032

Wilks' Lambda .8386   Chi Square 16.460   (5 d.f.)   Sig. .0056

public provider tend to view counseling for depression and spouse abuse and treatment for major mental illness as being more important. In comparison, those who would recommend a private provider view counseling for suicide and life changes as being more important (see Table 9).

IMPLICATIONS

The relative decline in public provider importance (and the corresponding increase in private provider importance) are among the most significant changes that have occurred in the mental health care market over the past several years. This, along with other factors, suggest the extent of competitiveness within the market and point to the need for sound marketing practices in order for a provider to be successful. However, little research that would be helpful to mental health care marketing managers has been reported. Findings from this study are a step toward filling this void.

Both unaided awareness of mental health providers and the ability to name a mental health provider that would be recommended to a friend are low, but both are significantly related to demographic characteristics. Awareness and recommendation of private providers are stronger among men and among higher income groups. Conversely, these factors relative to public providers are stronger among women and lower income groups. While age does not appear to strongly discriminate, those between the ages of 18 and 25 are more likely to recommend a public provider.

Table 8
MENTAL HEALTH CARE PROVIDERS THAT WOULD BE RECOMMENDED
TO FRIEND RELATED TO RELATIVE IMPORTANCE OF BENEFITS

	Public Providers	Private Providers
Total	36	62
Benefit	Imp. Rat.*	Imp. Rat*
Counseling for child/ teen beh. prob.	2.81	2.40
Counseling for teen suicide/depress.	2.72	2.37
Counseling for teen substance abuse	2.67	2.35
Counseling for adult substance abuse	2.67	2.60
Counseling for eating disorders	3.47	3.49
Counseling for stress	2.69	2.53
Counseling for anxiety	3.42	3.37
Counseling for depression	2.69	2.79
Counseling for suicide	3.02	2.69
Counseling for life changes	3.22	2.85
Counseling for child abuse	2.86	2.94
Counseling for spouse abuse	2.61	3.00
Treatment for major mental illness	3.11	3.35

* 1 = most important, 5 = least important

Table 9

DIFFERENCES IN IMPORTANCE OF BENEFITS
BETWEEN RECOMMENDED PROVIDER TYPE

	Canonical Loadings	Group Means Public Providers	Private Providers
Benefits			
Counseling for depression	-.4946	2.694	2.790
Counseling for suicide	.8937	3.028	2.694
Counseling for life changes	.5687	3.222	2.855
Counseling for spouse abuse	-.4690	2.611	3.000
Treatment for major mental illness	-.3768	3.111	3.355

Wilks' Lambda .8597   Chi Square 14.132 (5 d.f.) Sig. .0148

Note: Lower ratings indicate greater importance

The services offered by providers (or benefits sought by consumers) do not appear to be strongly related to either awareness or recommendation of providers. While the services tend to be viewed as equally important by both groups, there are some differences. Those "aware" of public providers view counseling for eating disorders, depression, and spouse abuse as being more important than do those "aware" of public providers. Conversely, those "aware" of private providers gave a slightly higher importance rating to counseling for life changes. Those who would recommend a public provider gave higher importance ratings to counseling for depression and spouse abuse and treatment for major mental illness. On the other hand, those who would recommend a private provider gave higher importance ratings for counseling for suicide and life changes.

This study was relatively narrow in scope and limited to one geographic market. Another limiting factor is that each of the provider types includes a variety of providers, some offer limited services while others offer a broader range of services. Certainly much more information is needed in order for mental health provider (both public and private) marketing managers to accomplish adequate planning. However, the findings have a number of management implications. The following are among the most salient implications.

1. Awareness, while somewhat higher for private providers, is low for both types of providers. Obviously, awareness is necessary before a consumer can make any considerations relative to a provider, including recommending that provider to a friend. A key consideration for all providers should be more and/or more effective marketing communications to increase awareness levels of potential service users.
2. The findings relative to demographics can be useful in planning and constructing these communications. Messages should reflect the appropriate demographic groups. In addition the messages should incorporate the important services/benefits. In addition, media that reaches the appropriate groups should be selected.
3. Managers of public service providers who wish to concentrate on their current market would concentrate on lower income,

younger, females. However, to broaden their market, effort should be directed to older, more affluent females as well as all males. The opposite would be appropriate for managers of private service providers.

4. The services/benefits that discriminate between the two service provider types tend to be among the less important of those measured. However, if a public service provider manager wishes to concentrate on her current market by promoting the provider's "strong" points, she would stress counseling for depression, spouse abuse, and eating disorders and treatment for major mental illness. To broaden the market, counseling for suicide and life changes might be stressed. Again, managers of private service providers would find the opposite appropriate.

REFERENCES

Ambrose, David M. and Linda Lennox (1988), "Strategic Market Positions for Mental Health Services," *Journal of Mental Health Administration*, 15 (Spring), 5-9.

Finn, David W. and Charles W. Lamb, Jr. (1986), "Hospital Benefit Segmentation," *Journal of Health Care Marketing*, 6 (Dec.), 26-33.

Frank, Ronald E., William F. Massey, and Donald G. Morrison (1965), "Bias in Multiple Discriminant Analysis," *Journal of Marketing Research* (August), 150-158.

Hoffman, E. Harvey and Stanley M. Nelson (1987), "The Successful Marketing of a Child and Adolescent Inpatient Unit in a Community Hospital," *Journal of Mental Health Administration*, 14 (Spring), 17-22.

Kotler, Philip and Roberta N. Clarke (1987), *Marketing for Health Care Organizations*. Englewood Cliffs, N.J.: Prentice-Hall, Inc.

Lim, Jeen-Su and Ron Zallocco (1988), "Determinant Attributes in Formulation of Attitudes Toward Four Health Care Systems," *Journal of Health Care Marketing*, 8 (June), 25-30.

Manderscheid, Ronald W. and Mary Anne Sonnenschein (1990), *Mental Health in the United States*, National Institute of Mental Health, DHHS Pub. No. (ADM) 90-1708, Washington, D.C.

Martin, John, (1988), "Problem Analysis: Application in the Development of Market Strategies for Health Care Organizations," *Journal of Health Care Marketing*, 8 (March), 5-16.

Perreault, William D., Douglas N. Behrman, and Gary M. Armstrong (1979), "Alternative Approaches for Interpretation of Multiple Discriminant Analysis," *Journal of Business Research*, (Vol. 7, 2), 151-173.

Stone, Terry R., William E. Warren, and Robert E. Stevens (1990), "Segmenting The Mental Health Market," *Journal of Health Care Marketing,* 10 (March), 65-69.

Woodside, Arch G. and Raymond Shinn (1988), "Customer Awareness and Preferences Toward Competing Hospital Services," *Journal of Health Care Marketing*, 8 (March), 39-47.

―――, Robert L. Nielsen, Fred Walters, and Gale D. Muller, (1988), "Preference Segmentation of Health Care Services: The Old-Fashioneds, Value Conscious, Affluents, and Professional Want-It-Alls," *Journal of Health Care Marketing*, 8 (June), 14-24.

Reports from the Field: Public Attitudes Toward People with Chronic Mental Illness: Executive Summary

The Robert Wood Johnson Foundation

Boston, Massachusetts

BACKGROUND

In the summer of 1989, The Robert Wood Johnson Foundation Program on Chronic Mental Illness[1] approached DYG, Inc., to conduct a major research project on American attitudes toward chronic mental illness and siting housing for people with chronic mental illness in communities and neighborhoods. The Robert Wood Johnson Foundation recognized that many communities have experienced resistance to all types of neighborhood sightings—the "Not In My Backyard" Phenomenon (NIMBY). The Program also wished to gain an in-depth understanding of the nature of resistance to and acceptance of housing facilities for people with chronic mental illness. The hope was that with this greater understanding, the Program would be better armed to overcome NIMBY.

Moreover, with virtually no recent national public opinion data available on attitudes toward chronic mental illness, the staff of the Program on Chronic Mental Illness wanted to explore general attitudes and perceptions.

Funding for this study was provided by: The Robert Wood Johnson Foundation, the American Psychiatric Association, the National Institute for Mental Health, and The PEW Charitable Trusts.

This article was prepared for The Robert Wood Johnson Foundation Program on Chronic Mental Illness, Boston, MA, and is reprinted with permission.

RESEARCH METHOD

In brief, the study findings are based on a survey of approximately 1,300 Americans, representative of the total population of adults 21 years of age and older. The survey was conducted by telephone between December 1 and December 11, 1989. In addition, two focus groups were conducted in Bala Cynwyd, Pennsylvania, and two were conducted in Columbus, Ohio, in September 1989. In-depth telephone interviews with 17 mental health opinion leaders were also conducted from September 19 to October 6, 1989. A more detailed discussion of the research and sampling methods employed is available on request.

KEY FINDINGS

1. The American public believes that the number of people with mental illness has increased in the past 20 years and that mental illness is a serious health problem in the U.S.
   * Fully seven in ten Americans (69%) believe that the incidence of mental illness has increased in the past 20 years — four in ten (41%) believe it has increased a lot.
   * Nine in ten (89%) describe mental illness as a serious problem in society today — 45% say it is a very serious problem.

2. An impressive number of Americans report personal experience with mental illness and mental health professionals.
   * One in three (31%) report that they or someone in their family have, at some time in their lives, sought the help of a psychiatrist or psychologist.
   * 14% of all Americans describe themselves or someone else close to them as currently having a mental illness.

3. Americans do not see themselves as "very well informed" about mental illness and say they should know a great deal more about it.
   * Only 25% describe themselves as "very well informed" about mental illness.

- Americans feel better informed about all other health problems tested — alcoholism (47%), cancer (43%), drug abuse (35%), heart disease (37%) and AIDS (30%).
- Six in ten (60%) say they should know more about mental illness.

4. Mass media is, far and away, the public' s primary source of information about mental illness, yet a minority find media coverage of mental illness believable.
    - Americans cite TV news and programs (87%), newspapers (76%), magazines (74%), and radio news and programs (73%) as their most frequent sources of information about mental illness. Far fewer cite family or friends (51%), mental health professionals (31%) or doctors (29%).
    - Yet only one in three (34%) describe TV, radio and newspaper stories about mental health as very believable — 61% describe them as "somewhat" believable.

5. Despite feeling that they do not know enough, Americans do believe the following important things about mental illness.
    - Anyone can become mentally ill (74%).
    - Mental illness can be cured (74%).
    - Most people with mental illness can, with treatment, get well and return to productive lives (54%).
    - Keeping up a normal life in the community will help a person with mental illness get better (53%).
    - Having a mental illness is no different from having any other kind of illness (43%).

6. Two in three (65%) believe there is still a lot of stigma attached to mental illness.

7. Americans believe that mental illness can be caused by physical disturbances (such as chemical imbalances in the brain (91%)), by environmental conditions (such as daily stress (90%)) or by alcoholism or drug abuse (93%).

8. The "Not In My Backyard" Phenomenon (NIMBY) emerges as widespread and a great barrier to opportunities for people

with mental illness. Opposition to the siting of any type of facility appears to be fairly widespread.

- Over one in ten (14%) say that their neighborhood has opposed some type of facility (ranging from a school, hospital, drug treatment center or garbage dump) in the past five years. And half of those who said that there has been opposition in the past five years indicated that this opposition was successful in stopping plans for siting facilities in their neighborhood.

9. It is quite apparent that all facilities are not created equal.

Respondents were asked to use a six-point scale to rate the acceptability of 18 types of facilities that could be placed in their neighborhood. Once data were tabulated, it became clear that three distinct tiers of acceptability exist.

- The first tier consists of several facilities that are most welcome by community residents. These facilities include: a school, a day care center, a nursing home, a hospital, and a medical clinic.
- The second tier is composed of facilities that received a mixed review: a group home for the mentally retarded, a homeless shelter, an alcohol rehabilitation center, and a drug treatment center.
- The third or last tier consists of facilities that most residents absolutely do not want in their community. These facilities include: a shopping mall, a group home for AIDS patients, a factory, a garbage landfill, and a prison.

10. Facilities for people with chronic mental illness are not among the more acceptable facilities.

- Eight different descriptions of facilities for persons with chronic mental illness were examined in this study. The ratings for most of these facilities fall at the lower end of the second tier of acceptable facilities.

11. While acceptance and support of siting facilities in neighborhoods vary by demographic groups, income is the single best predictor of opposition to facilities — opposers (NIMBYs) are more likely to be in affluent neighborhoods.

- As noted earlier, over one in ten (14%) said that their neighborhood had acted to oppose a facility in the past five years. However, over two in ten (21%) of those with a household income of $50,000 and over say that their neighborhood has been involved in opposing a facility during the past five years.
- Furthermore, a similar pattern emerges when the acceptability level of specific facilities is examined — the acceptability of neighborhood facilities decreases as income increases. That is, lower (under $15,000) and moderate ($15-24,999) household income groups are more accepting than affluent households (annual household income of $50,000 or more) of all types of neighborhood facilities.
- These NIMBYs also tend to be:
  - Male
  - Well-educated
  - Professionals
  - Married
  - Homeowners
  - Living in large cities or suburbs of large cities

12. Social values help explain the NIMBY Phenomenon.

    Respondents were given a battery of questions excerpted from the DYG Environmental Scanning Program,[2] an ongoing national study of America's changing social values and "NIMBYs" are very much in keeping with trends in America toward the following characteristics:
    - Pessimistic about the future.
    - Fearful of taking chances in their lives. In a sense, they are risk averse.
    - Competitive.
    - Darwinistic, believing in individual mastery.
    - And less tolerant of differences.

13. Finally, NIMBYs' beliefs about mental illness are less hopeful than those of the general population. They are less likely to believe that:
    - Anyone can become mentally ill.
    - Most people with mental illness can get well and return to productive lives.

For more information contact:

Diane D. Barry
Communications Director
Robert Wood Johnson Foundation
Program on Chronic Mental Illness
74 Fenwood Road
Boston, MA 02115
(617) 738-7774

NOTES

1. The Program on Chronic Mental Illness is a national demonstration project of the Robert Wood Johnson Foundation. With a five-year grant, it is establishing a comprehensive mental health system, including rehabilitation and housing, in nine urban areas: Austin, Texas; Baltimore, Maryland; Charlotte, North Carolina; Cincinnati, Ohio; Columbus, Ohio; Denver, Colorado; Honolulu, Hawaii; Philadelphia, Pennsylvania; and Toledo, Ohio.

2. The DYG Environmental Scanning Program is an annual tracking study of American social values that identifies trends in public lifestyles and values.

Stakeholder Perspectives: Divergent Views of the Mental Health System

Teri A. Kline
Greg Carlson

BACKGROUND

This study evolved from the desire of the Alabama Department of Mental Health and Mental Retardation and the Alabama State Mental Illness Planning Council created under Public Law 99-660 to solicit input from important stakeholders in the mental health system in preparation for the continuing revision of the department's planning efforts.

This is not the first study to look at various subgroups within a mental health system to determine their perceptions. One notable study in New York questioned family members of the mentally ill on a variety of topics including attitudes and satisfaction related to

Teri A. Kline, MBA, is affiliated with Auburn University at Montgomery. Greg Carlson, MBA, is Director, Planning and Research, Alabama Department of Mental Health and Mental Retardation.

treatment such as type of program, satisfaction with staff and inter-action with mental health professionals (Grosser, 1988). In two studies (Lefley, 1989 and Wahl and Harman, 1989) the related is-sue of family stigma is studied.

METHODOLOGY

A mail survey was distributed to appropriate stakeholders in the Alabama mental health system including primary consumers, fam-ily members of the mentally ill, advocates, state institution pro-viders, community program providers and public or private hospi-tals. This study analyzes the 383 usable questionnaires returned by persons identifying themselves as primary consumers, family mem-bers or advocates.

A survey questionnaire was developed by members of the Alli-ance for the Mentally Ill of Alabama, primary consumers, Auburn University at Montgomery, community providers, and the Alabama Department of Mental Health and Mental Retardation. The survey explored the stakeholder's perceptions on a variety of issues includ-ing missing or weak elements in the Mental Health System, family education and support issues, discharge planning and follow-up and perception of access to mental health services and information.

MISSING/WEAK ELEMENTS IN THE SYSTEM

Three broad areas were surveyed in this section of the question-naire including facility issues, program issues and issues concern-ing facilitation of return to the community. Respondents were asked to rank the most important missing elements and weakest existing elements in the current continuum of care (Table 1).

The elements dealing with facilities or the distribution of services included housing, residential alternatives, institutions and institu-tion/community coordination. All three groups (consumers, family members and advocates) had similar perceptions on the residential alternatives element with on the average half of the respondents indicating this is a missing element. Fewer persons (one in six) felt that institutions were a weak or missing link, while on the average one fourth of the group saw a need for more institution/community

TABLE 1
MISSING/ WEAK ELEMENTS IN SYSTEM

Elements	Consumers N= 121	Family N= 148	Advocates N= 114
	%	%	%
Distribution/ Facility Issues			
Housing	33	42	52
Residential Alternatives*	46	50	48
Institution/ Community Coordination	21	24	25
Institutions	18	16	17
Product/ Program Issues			
Crisis Stabilization***	45	74	81
Case Management*	40	56	57
Family Education	34	30	26
Issues Concerning Facilitation of Return To Community			
Employment Opportunities	48	43	48
Vocational Rehabilitation	31	36	28
Day Treatment**	40	12	21
Outpatient Treatment***	31	19	12
Psychological/Social Rehabilitation**	21	37	31
Self Help***	35	16	16
Medical/ Dental Assistance**	25	14	12

* Difference Significant at .1
** Difference Significant at .05
***Difference Significant at .01

coordination. The only area in this group where the consumers, family and advocates differed significantly was in their perception of housing alternatives. Consumers were less likely to see this as a problem (33%) while slightly over half of the advocates see a problem in this area (52%). Family members fell somewhere between these two groups with 42% of them seeing housing alternatives as a weak or missing element.

Programmatic issues brought more differences between the three groups. The most significant difference was in the perception of crisis stabilization programs. Advocates (81%) and family members (74%) were more likely to see this as a missing link in the system

than consumers (45%). Another noteworthy difference is in perceptions about case management. Again, advocates (57%) and family
members (56%) were more likely than consumers (40%) to see case
management services as a weak or missing element. There was only
a slight difference in perceptions about family education, with consumers (34%) more likely to see this as a problem than either family
members (30%) or advocates (26%).

Seven of the issues listed on the survey dealt with facilitation of
return to the community. The most commonly listed problem for all
three groups was employment opportunities. Consumers and advocates (both 48%) saw this as slightly more of a problem than did
family members (43%). Across the board, another commonly
ranked problem was vocational rehabilitation. On the average one
in three respondents ranked this as a key issue. Some differences in
perceptions arise in several of the other issues concerning return to
the community. Consumers were more likely (40%) than family
members (26%) or advocates (21%) to see a need in the area of day
treatment. Consumers were also more likely to rank outpatient
treatment (31%), self-help groups (35%) and medical and dental
assistance (25%) as a problem than family and advocates were. On
the other hand, family members were the most likely of the three
groups to list the need for psychological/social rehabilitation (37%)
as a weak link in the system.

When questioned about specific areas of the delivery system including care for the homeless, adolescents, children, rural residents, elderly, or minorities, there were few differences in perceptions (Table 2). Overall there was a higher perception that
improvement was needed in care for the homeless. The only significant difference between the three groups was in the perception of
care for minorities with consumers seeing this as a bigger problem.

FAMILY EDUCATION AND SUPPORT

Generally speaking, family members and advocates saw more
need for improvement in family education and support issues than
did the consumers (Table 3). Significant differences surface in education and information improvement issues. Family members (32%)
and advocates (31%) were more likely than consumers (19%) to

suggest increasing family education and training. Likewise, these two groups were more willing to suggest involving and communicating with the family. Although not perceived as a major issue overall, family members and advocates suggested the use of media and getting information to the community more often than did consumers.

DISCHARGE PLANNING

Two areas surfaced as issues in the discharge planning and follow-up programs: communication issues and program improvement issues (Table 4). As far as communication is concerned, advocates are far more likely (25%) than consumers (14%) or family members (15%) to see the need for better communication between institutions and Mental Health Centers.

Program improvement issues such as better follow-up, better case management and improved family support were more likely to be suggested by family members and advocates while teaching independent living skills was popular with consumers.

TABLE 2
SPECIALTY SERVICE DELIVERY SYSTEM
IMPROVEMENT ISSUES

Issues	Consumers N= 121	Family N= 148	Advocates N= 114
	%	%	%
Homeless	28	22	18
Adolescent	13	14	15
Children	8	13	11
Rural	11	11	14
Geriatric	7	4	4
Minority *	8	2	2

* Difference Significant at .05

TABLE 3

FAMILY EDUCATION/SUPPORT ISSUES

Issues	Consumers N= 121	Family N= 148	Advocates N= 114
	%	%	%
Group Support			
Increase Family Therapy Support Groups	15	18	18
Get Churches/Other Agencies Involved	4	4	6
Work With Advocacy Groups	0	4	6
More Funding	4	5	8
Education/ Information Improvement			
Increase Family Education Training*	19	32	31
Involve/ Communicate With Family***	12	25	29
Use Media/ Get Information to Community**	2	9	8

* Difference Significant at .1
** Difference Significant at .05
*** Difference Significant at .01

TABLE 4
DISCHARGE PLANNING/ FOLLOW-UP ISSUES

Issues	Consumers N=121	Family N=148	Advocates N=114
	%	%	%
Communication			
Better Communication Between Institutions and Community Mental Health Centers*	14	15	25
Better Communication With Clients	4	5	4
Program Improvement Issues			
Better Follow-up**	9	26	27
Better Case Management**	6	16	23
Improved Family Support	7	13	11
Teaching Independent Living Skills***	9	2	4

* Difference Significant at .1
** Difference Significant at .05
*** Difference Significant at .01

ACCESS ISSUES

Respondents were asked how to improve information access as well as service access in the mental health system. Suggestions for improving information access fell into three broad areas: external communications, intra-system communication and system improvements (Table 5). There were only slight differences in perceptions between the consumers, family members and advocates. The biggest problem across the groups was seen as a need for external communications such as educating the community, publicity and advertising. The next most common perceived need was in the intra-system communication for a centralized referral service communication network with advocates and family members listing this more often than consumers did. Other intra-system suggestions included communication between agencies and case management.

Some respondents indicated ways to improve information access would include system improvements such as staff training, educating mental health professionals on available services and more funding.

Suggestions for improving system access fell into two broad categories: facility issues and staff/management issues (Table 6). There were no significant differences between the three groups on facility issues such as better accessibility, more outpatient programs and better indigent care.

The only significant difference in this section appears under the suggestion for more staff, with almost twice as many advocates (27%) suggesting this solution as did family members (15%) or consumers (13%). Other methods listed by the three groups include reduce waiting time/"red tape," more efficient case management, better quality of staff and educating the community. There were only slight differences in the perception for these solutions between the groups.

CONCLUSION

This study was designed to provide an initial description of the need areas in the Alabama system as determined by various stakeholder groups. A future more detailed survey is anticipated to compare alternative strategies for meeting these needs.

TABLE 5
HOW TO IMPROVE INFORMATION ACCESS

Elements	Consumers N= 121	Family N= 148	Advocates N= 114
	%	%	%
External Communications			
Educate Community	24	35	31
Publicize/ Advertise	23	27	22
Intra-System Communication			
Centralize Referral Service Communication	11	17	21
Between Agencies	3	4	3
Case Management	2	2	5
System Improvements			
Improve/ Train Staff	8	10	9
Educate MH Professionals on Services Available	4	2	5
More Funding/ Staff	4	4	8

TABLE 6
HOW TO IMPROVE SYSTEM ACCESS

Issues	Consumers N= 121	Family N= 148	Advocates N= 114
	%	%	%
Facility Issues			
Better Accessibility/Provide Transportation	12	9	13
More Outpatient Programs	2	5	8
Better Indigent Care	2	5	4
Staff/ Management Issues			
More Staff*	13	15	27
Reduce Waiting/ Less Red Tape	6	11	10
More Efficient Case Management	9	10	16
Better Quality Staff	10	8	11
Educate Community	8	5	3

* Difference Significant at .05

While this study reflects the needs in one state, it, along with the previous studies mentioned provide a starting point for mental health systems and providers in assessing the needs from a "customer" perspective. To the extent that many of the issues addressed are universal problems in state mental health systems, this study can be used as a guideline for identifying the weak or missing elements in the system. It can also be used as a basis for planning family and support programs and addressing problems in discharge and follow-up. To the extent that information and system access are problems, available programs cannot be utilized to their potential. This study gives an indication of access problems in the mental health system. Planning in the state mental health system must include the perspectives of the stakeholders being served by and serving the system. Identifying and targeting the multiple markets in any system is the essential starting point in the planning process.

SOURCES

Grosser, Rene C. and Phyllis Vine, "Family Member Survey Summary of Results," Presentation at the Alliance for the Mentally Ill of the State of New York Sixth Educational Conference, Buffalo, New York, October 9, 1988.

Lefley, Harriet P., "Family Burden and Family Stigma in Major Mental Illness," *American Psychologist*, March 1989, pp. 556-559.

Wahl, Otto F. and Charles R. Harman, "Family Views of Stigma," *Schizophrenia Bulletin*, Vol. 15, No. 1, pp. 131-138.

REFERRAL AND SECONDARY RESOURCE MARKETS

Using Demographic Segmentation Variables to Identify Financial Donors for Mental Health Services

Ronald E. Milliman
L. W. Turley

SUMMARY. The purpose of this study was to explore the possible relationships between the demographic characteristics of potential donors to nonprofit, philanthropic organizations and their perceptions of the three most pressing human care needs with analytical emphasis on those who identified mental health issues, in particular, as pressing.

There were five demographic variables used in this specific study; they were gender, race, age, number of children in the family, and the number of adults in the family.

None of these specific demographic variables yielded significant results. Hence, based upon the limited scope of this study, demographics did not appear to be particularly useful in segmenting this market.

Ronald Milliman, PhD, is Professor of Marketing and Lou Turley, DBA, is Assistant Professor of Marketing at Western Kentucky University, Bowling Green, KY 42101.

INTRODUCTION

As nonprofit mental health care centers enter the 1990's, they clearly face a variety of tough challenges. Direct federal funding, since 1982, has been cut substantially, in excess of 25 percent; and based upon a survey of 104 mental health centers, nearly 50 percent reported their financial status had steadily deteriorated since 1981 (Okin 1984, p. 1119). A study of community mental health centers conducted over a three-year period throughout 15 different states found that centers were even more dependent on the states today than they were on the federal government in the past (Larsen 1986).

Government support for nonprofit services continues to decrease, and competition between service providers for donations from individuals is increasing. Demand for nonprofit and public services such as mental health, however, is also clearly increasing.

Nonprofit services are then caught between the proverbial rock and a hard place. The supply of funds is drying up while demand is increasing at a rapid rate. Centers have responded to this situation in various ways. Some have been forced to reduce staffing, increase clinician caseloads, cut back overall levels of services, and centralize their operations through the closing of satellite centers. Others have attempted to offset decreases in governmental support through more efficient billing and collection, development of management information systems, and establishment of for-profit (as opposed to nonprofit) corporations, and by changing the balance of service modalities and patient populations from those that fail to generate fees to those that do (Okin 1984, p. 1120).

Another vitally important area that could contribute to the overall solution to the problem of funding mental health care and other similar nonprofit organizations is through more effective and efficient marketing to potential donors. However, understanding the wants and needs of the organizations' many significant publics (i.e., clients, potential donors, etc.) is critical to the successful implementation of the marketing concept. Too many nonprofit service providers, including mental health organizations, focus on their products and services rather than the client and other significant publics including current and potential donors (Andreasen 1982). As a result of such an emphasis, nonprofit organizations have a tendency to use undifferentiated strategies aimed at the "average" or largest segment of donors (Lamb 1987). Since few people are "average," by definition this strategy fails to satisfy almost everyone.

Consequently, a segmentation strategy appears to be warranted in this situation. Segmentation allows marketers to break down the total market for a good or service into smaller and more homogeneous groups. Distinct strategies can then be developed specifically for each of the targeted segments, increasing the effectiveness of marketing campaigns.

In a similar manner, segmenting the potential donor market and targeting individual prospective contributors to mental health organizations would appear to be especially appropriate. For instance, an examination of some donation figures shows private individuals donated 83.1% of all philanthropical giving in the U.S. in 1988, but they only accounted for 69.5% of all giving to health-related organizations (Giving USA 1988). Individual donations are supporting other philanthropical causes to a greater degree than they are health in general and mental health specifically. Therefore, identifying and targeting individuals interested in mental health issues should result in increased donations and larger war chests to use to combat the problem.

AN EXAMINATION OF RELATED LITERATURE

Most authors suggest four dimensions for segmenting markets: geographic segmentation, psychographic segmentation, demographic segmentation, and behavioral segmentation. According to Kotler, of these four broad segmentation approaches, demographic variables appear to be promising segmentation tools for nonprofit marketers.

Several researchers have explored demographic differences in donation behavior with some interesting results. Edmundson (1986) observed that age does seem to influence donation behavior. People aged 35 to 64 are most likely to donate, and those from 50 to 64 give the most of all. The 30 to 35 age group, however, gives very little. Edmundson believes that younger donors are skeptical and tend not to give unless they know exactly where the money is going.

Harvey (1990) explored the use of benefit segmentation in non-

profit situations and uncovered some interesting demographic varia-
tions. He argues that females and nonwhites are likely to be part of
what he identified as the manager segment. This group is considered to be more interested in the operations of the fund raiser rather
than its aims. This group gave the highest percentage of income and
gave because "it felt good." Guy and Patton (1989) disagree with
the use of gender as a segmentation variable and believe that helping
behavior is unrelated to gender. However, given the shift of attitudes of blacks toward mental health issues, there is some reason
to believe race could be a promising donor segmentation factor
(Lawrence, 1987).

The question of can demographic variables be used to identify
and segment the donor market is the essence of this present empiri-
cal study which is discussed in the remainder of this paper.

THE PRESENT STUDY

This study explored possible demographic differences among donors interested in different nonprofit causes. The research question
addressed here is can selected demographics be used to differentiate
donors that are interested in supporting nonprofit mental health organizations from those interested in supporting other causes?

The Sample

In order to investigate this issue, a questionnaire was developed
and administered to a sample of potential donors. The sample consisted of all the employees of several large firms located in a city in
the southeast region of the United States. Each of the firms was
selected specifically because it participates regularly in an annual
fund raiser for a well-known, national nonprofit organization (The
United Way). There were a total of 625 subjects in the resulting
sample.

The Questionnaire

Based upon a combination of researcher judgment and the results
of a pre-test, the questionnaire provided a list of eighteen potential
human care service needs. The subjects were, then, asked to identify the three most pressing human care service needs from this list

with a nineteenth alternative of listing their own most pressing human care service needs. The eighteen listed causes from which the respondent could select the three most pressing were:

1. Alcohol and drug abuse
2. Child abuse
3. Homelessness
4. The physically disabled
5. The poor and needy
6. Mental health
7. Crime
8. Spouse abuse
9. Hunger
10. Emergency services
11. Environmental issues
12. Unemployment
13. Teenage pregnancy
14. Child day-care services
15. Services for the elderly
16. Illiteracy
17. Youth development services
18. Family counseling

In addition, based on the research cited earlier in the literature review section of this paper, the questionnaire also asked respondents to identify their status on several demographic variables. These variables were gender, race, number of children in the family, the number of adults in the family, and age.

Analytical Procedures Used

Since some of the demographic variables can be classified as metric variables while others were nonmetric, different statistical procedures were used to examine the relationships, if any, between demographics and donor interest in various perceived pressing issues in general and mental health issues specifically. Gender and race, for instance, are nonmetric variables since the associated numbers are arbitrarily assigned to groups to represent a category (Hair et al. 1979). Therefore, chi-square analysis was used to test the differences between those identifying mental health as a pressing issue from those who did not.

In contrast, the number of children in the family, the number of adults in the family, and age are all metric data since the variables have constant units of measurement (Hair et al. 1979). Therefore, these variables were examined using discriminant analysis, since this procedure is used to examine the relationship between metric independent variables and nonmetric dependent variables (Hair et al. 1979).

RESULTS OF THE STUDY

Out of the 625 responses, only 14% listed mental health as one of the three issues they considered particularly pressing. Thus, 86% of the respondents did not identify mental health as one of their perceived pressing human needs.

The results of the chi-square analysis for gender and race are presented in Table I. In both cases, the differences between donors listing mental health as a pressing need from those that did not list it as a pressing need were insignificant. Neither variable appears to be a good predictor of behavior in this case.

Stepwise discriminant analysis was used to distinguish between donor perceptions of pressing needs, the number of children in the family, the number of adults in the family, and age. Since stepwise discriminant analysis is designed to find the set of variables which maximizes the discriminant power as defined by some criteria (SPSSX Users Guide 1983), the combinations of variables which minimize the overall Wilks lambda were sought as this criteria.

However, based on this criterion, only one variable, age, entered into the solution. The inclusion of either the number of children in the family or the number of adults in the family would have increased the overall Wilks lambda. The summary table for this action is presented in Table II.

The method for validation consisted of forming a classification table which indicates the percentage of cases which would be classified correctly using the discriminant function. The results of this classification are presented in Table III. The overall percentage of

Table I
RESULTS OF CHI-SQUARE ANALYSIS

VARIABLE	CHI-SQUARE	D.F.	SIGNIFICANCE
gender	.86810	1	n.s.
race	1.70364	2	n.s.

Table II
Summary of the Discriminate Analysis

Eigen Value	Canonical Correlation	Wilks Lambda	Chi-Square	D.F.	Significance
0.01770	0.1318852	.9826063	4.7288	1	0.0297

Table III
Classification Results

Predicted Group Membership

Actual Group	1	2
1	63.4%	36.6%
2	56.3%	43.7%

cases classified correctly was 60.89%. Hair et al. (1979) recommends the proportional chance criterion as the test of significance.

In this situation, where group sizes were 14% and 86%, respectively, the proportional chance criterion is 78.92%. Since only 60.89% were correctly classified using these demographic variables, the results are insignificant. Hair et al. (1979) recommends that classification accuracy be at least 25% more likely than by chance alone, which did not occur in this instance.

CONCLUSIONS, LIMITATIONS, AND RECOMMENDATIONS

The purpose of this study was to explore the relationship between the demographic characteristics of potential donors and their identification of various pressing human needs in general and mental health issues specifically. The five demographic variables used in this particular study were gender, race, age, number of children in the family, and the number of adults in the family.

None of these specific demographic variables yielded significant results. Hence, the specific five demographic variables used in this study do not appear to be particularly useful in segmenting this market.

This study, however, has a few obvious limitations. The questionnaires were all self-administered; therefore, the exact interpretation of each question was subject to the respondents' perceptions of their wording. In addition, the sample was not a random selection of persons in a defined population, but rather it was, in effect, a convenience sample. Hence, the reader must be cautioned against generalizing these results beyond the relatively narrow scope of this specific study. Finally, the five demographic variables examined, while selected based upon previous research, proved to be quite limiting.

Future research in this area should either explore additional and/ or different demographic variables, including their cross relationships and interactions. Additionally, other approaches (singularly or in combination) could be employed, such as psychographic segmentation, behavioral segmentation, or perhaps even geographic segmentation. It might be very worthwhile to look more specifically at the present and potential donor status of those persons who have directly and/or indirectly received assistance from a mental health organization, including their friends and relatives. For instance, a survey conducted by the Media Research Bureau of the University of Missouri-Columbia reported that 31.9 percent of 1,012 persons residing in the state of Missouri responded affirmatively to the question: "Have you or a member of your immediate family ever been treated for mental illness?" Thus, these persons could possibly comprise a segment of potential donors. Certainly, it would be reasonable to assume this client segment is concerned about the state of mental health and the stigma associated with it. This assumption is further reinforced by a survey of 486 members of the National Alliance of Mental Health conducted by Wahl and Harman (1989). Could it be that members of this Alliance, for instance, represent a sizable segment of potential donors, given their interest and concern?

REFERENCES

Andreasen, Alan R. (1982), "Nonprofits: Check Your Attention to Customers," *Harvard Business Review*, 60 (No. 3): 105-110.

Edmondson, Brad (1986), "Who Gives to Charity?," *American Demographics*, 8 (November): 44-49.

Giving USA 1988. 1988 Annual Report, New York: American Association of Fund Raising Council.

Guy, Bonnie S. and Wesley E. Patton (1989), "The Marketing of Altruistic Causes: Understanding Why People Help," *The Journal of Consumer Marketing*, 6 (No. 1): 19-30.

Hair, Joseph F., Rolph E. Anderson, Ronald L. Tatham and Bernie J. Grablowsky (1979). *Multivariate Data Analysis*, Tulsa, Oklahoma: Petroleum Publishing Company.

Harvey, James W. (1990), "Benefit Segmentation for Fund Raisers," *Journal of the Academy of Marketing Science*, 18 (No. 1), 77-86.

Lamb, Charles W. (1987), "Public Sector Marketing is Different," *Business Horizons*, 30 (No. 4), 56-60.

Larsen, Judith K. (1986), "Local Mental Health Agencies in Transition," *American Behavioral Scientist*, 30 (No. 2), 174-187.

Lawrence, Gary E. (1987), "Attitudes of Black Adults Toward Community Mental Health Centers," *Hospital and Community Psychiatry*, 38 (No. 10), 1100-1105.

Okin, Robert L. (1984), "How Community Mental Health Centers are Coping," *Hospital and Community Psychiatry*, 35 (No. 11), 1118-1129.

SPSSX Users Guide (1983). SPSS Inc., New York: McGraw-Hill Book Company.

Wahl, Otto. F., Charles R. Harman (1989), "Family Views of Stigma," *Schizophrenia Bulletin*, 15 (No. 1), 131-138.

Employing Local Norms to Identify Potential Referral Agents of Mental Health Care Clients

Ronald L. Coulter
R. Stephen Parker
Mary K. Coulter

As the population of the United States moves toward the next century, concern for the mental health of our population will become even more important. Several factors will become important including: (1) political and economic forces as they influence the relative concern given to social issues, and (2) the large numbers of "baby boomers" who will be moving into their 50's and may demand a higher level of social services. As mental health service providers attempt to plan for the future they must be cognizant of these issues as well as the importance of local social norms regarding the perceptions of mental health issues and treatment.

"Local norms" (Cox et al. 1976) refers to both local community and subcultural standards for behavior and deviance. Local attitudes are recognized as important indicators of the types of referrals received by community mental health centers. As Cox and others (1976, p. 902) have stated, ". . . it is only after people's behavior has become problematic for themselves, their family, or their associates that they are referred to the mental health agency." Based on

Ronald L. Coulter and R. Stephen Parker are Associate Professors of Marketing at Southwest Missouri State University. Mary K. Coulter is Associate Professor of Management at Southwest Missouri State University. Address correspondence to the authors at: Southwest Missouri State University, 901 S. National Street, Springfield, MO 65804-0094.

this assumption a two-staged problem exists for the mental health care marketer. First, the marketer must identify those individuals in the community who are the likely referral agents, and second, the marketer must understand the attitudes and general views of those local referral agents toward those mental health problems considered to be problematic.

From a marketing perspective the service provider must identify the local community opinion leaders who serve as referral agents to understand their attitudes toward a variety of issues related to community mental health norms. By understanding the local norms the marketer can match service offerings to individual community needs. The purpose of the present study is to demonstrate a methodology to examine the attitudes and perceptions of several types of referral agents in local communities where mental health care facilities exist.

LITERATURE REVIEW

Market Potential

The need for mental health care services is very evident. A national survey (*Time* 1986) indicated that fully 20% of the adult population in the United States is mentally troubled at any given time. It is further estimated that between 29% and 38% of the adult population will experience at least one psychiatric problem in their lifetimes (Ahmed and Viswanathan 1984). As our population ages, more and more of these problems will likely manifest themselves in the form of behaviors unacceptable to local community standards.

The most prevalent problems found in the 1984 *Time* study are Anxiety with 8.3% of the population being affected and 23% of these cases receiving treatment, Alcohol and Drugs with 6.4% of the population affected and 18% of these cases treated, Depression affecting 6.0% of the population and 32% of the cases treated, and Schizophrenia affecting 1.0% of the population with 53% of these cases receiving treatment (*Time* 1986).

One of the more interesting findings relates to the fact that while many people suffer from "mental health" problems, only a small percentage of those people actually receive any type of professional treatment. As such, it would appear that many potential clients have not been referred for treatment thus exposing a potential gap in the marketing channel. While it is obvious that a significant number of people do have mental health problems, it is also likely that many of these individuals do not yet have problems severe enough in terms of "local norms" to require treatment.

Stigmas

Literature relating to the field of mental health or mental illness strongly indicates the general public has a negative perception of those individuals who have had problems severe enough to seek or require treatment. According to Page (1974), there is considerable evidence to confirm the existence of a very negative image of the "mental patient." Piner and Kahle (1984) also reported that the label of mental illness is stigmatizing even in the absence of bizarre behavior. Stensrud and Stensrud (1980) noted that there was ample evidence to demonstrate an oppressive stigma that is attached to psychiatric hospitalization. Stensrud's assertion may be applicable to more than just those who are actually hospitalized.

Because many mental health professionals are called "doctors" and treatment may include drugs of various types (Farina et al. 1978), mental health problems are viewed by outsiders as a physical illness. In fact, most people seek help for mental health problems from medical doctors than from mental health specialists (Kohler and Corrigan 1983-84). Several factors must be considered by marketers when dealing with these negative perceptions. In communities where the public skeptically views a person who seeks help from a mental health professional (doctor) a stigma must be overcome. Further, even though the public may not actually discriminate against the mental patient, the belief that discrimination exists may be self-fulfilling. As such, a person who does not need or require treatment for a specific problem would still be hesitant to seek out the services of a community mental health center. The importance of confidentiality in dealing with patients might help to alleviate the patient's concern that the community would imply that he or she did have a mental health problem and which would evoke the responsive stigmas. Once again the local norms of the community and the supportiveness of local referral agents would be of primary concern in the marketing of the mental health center.

Local Norms

The lack of a clear, general understanding of the term "mental health" and the public's general negative predisposition to the topic likely varies from locale to locale. As Cox et al. (1976) has stated, the only relevant way to deal with the issues previously discussed is at the local level. The degree of understanding or misunderstanding, and the related stigmas attached to mental health issues are likely correlated with the local communities level of social education (Ahmed and Viswanathan 1984 and Piner and Kahle 1984). During the 1960 to 1970 era mental health propaganda became prevalent in our society (Farina et al. 1978). As a result of the increase in information, researchers concluded that popular mental health attitudes were changing for the better (Olmsted and Durham 1976). Two diverse views were presented on this predicted change of attitudes. The negative view held that the negative stigmas were based on strong cultural beliefs and were therefore not likely to be influenced by the external forces of educational and/or promotional campaigns (Olmsted and Durham 1976). One study used to support this position indicated that while mental health propaganda had the tendency to be effective, the attitude changes are so small that the results held little practical importance.

The more positive view of the issues assumes that because the general public is uncertain as to what "mental health" really is, the public is inclined to change its views when provided with new information. If this view is correct, the more information the individual receives the more likely the individual would be to show greater attitude changes. Farina et al. (1978) argues that beliefs about mental health appear to change because society's perceptions are at least partially determined by the amount of information presented by mental health agencies. Olmsted and Durham (1976) presents a similar positive view by indicating that a better understanding of mental health will come from the more enlightened opinions of younger people and those exposed to more information. Again, depending upon the amount of information received by each community, local norms will play an important role in the design of a mental health center's marketing strategy.

Gate Keepers as Referral Agents

Often community gatekeepers are the opinion leaders in the community. As such, it is logical that a two-step communication approach for reaching local referral agents might be advantageous. DeMello (1983-1984) suggested a simple approach for marketing mental health agencies that would employ the following 4 steps:

1. Identify all major target groups for planning and service development.
2. Set criteria for selection and prioritization of key target groups.
3. Analyze target groups, select, and prioritize key groups.
4. Develop a specific program for each key target group.

DeMello noted that such an approach is a departure from most health care planning methodologies which he described as "inside out" approaches. The more common "inside out" approach occurs when the mental health care provider determines what services it will offer and then attempts to sell them to the market. DeMello's 4-step model is based on the marketing concept philosophy of determining what the local community needs and then attempting to develop mental health services to satisfy the market's needs.

Two studies conducted in 1980 and 1981 concluded that gate-keepers do exist and they can be divided into several categories each having varying levels of influence in their respective communities (Kohler and Corrigan 1983-1984). The findings of the 1980 study indicated that Psychiatrist/Psychologist was most recommended (28.6%), followed by Physician (27.8%), Mental Health Agency (21.9%), Clergy (9.3%), Hospital (2.8%), and Other (5.6%). The 1981 study varied only slightly. In this study, Psychiatrist/Psychologist were given the highest recommendation (33.7%) followed by Mental Health Agency (25.7%), Physician (22.3%), Clergy (15.9%), and Other (2.3%). A partial explanation for the differences between the two studies is that the 1980 study used an open-ended questionnaire while the 1981 study used a multiple choice questionnaire.

The literature also indicates that most referrals to community mental health agencies take place only when problems or concerns are experienced by family, friends, and local institutions which might include the work place or religious institutions (Cox et al. 1976). Generally such referrals occur only after the behavior has become problematic. While each individual's problem has a more micro solution, the determination of how the general public perceives "mental illness" is a macro problem for each community and thus a more difficult problem to deal with.

Given the problems which have been examined, several conclusions may be drawn from the literature. First the general public does not appear to have a clearly defined view of the term "mental health," but rather a general negative feeling toward the term. It has also been suggested that this lack of understanding may be due in part to a lack of education about mental illness and with continued education the stigma associated with the term may be lessened (Ahmed and Viswanathan 1984 and Piner and Kahle 1984). Questions which remain include, how do local mental health agencies reach more of those individuals who have problems severe enough to require treatment, and how can local agencies overcome any negative perceptions of mental illness and its likely carryover to mental health facilities?

The resulting implication of the literature is that community mental health centers must understand the local community's norms through those people who are the appropriate opinion leaders, and consequentially the gatekeepers to success. If Morrison et al. (1977) study indicating that future professionals may reflect a decreased acceptance of the value of psychodiagnostic assessment, then certainly community mental health centers will face decreasing referrals by local community professionals. The task is to both understand and educate the general population and the gatekeeper target markets about the value of services offered by local community mental health centers. The remainder of this article presents a methodology designed to examine the attitudes and perceptions of local referral agents in a large midwestern community having a relatively new mental health care center. Using this methodology, local norms and education levels were assessed to develop appropriate service delivery and educational marketing strategies.

RESEARCH OBJECTIVES

The objectives of the present study were:

1. To determine if significant differences in referral agent attitudes toward mental health care service providers exist in local markets.
2. To determine if significant differences in referral agent perceptions of local community problems exist.
3. To determine whether local referral agents would express significant differences in whom they would personally seek for help if they were in need of mental health care help.
4. To determine if any consistent patterns exist across the three research objectives previously presented, which would be useful in the development of an effective strategic marketing plan based on local community norms.

METHODOLOGY

Sample Development

Using the information found in the literature review, it was determined that a survey would be developed for use with a local SMSA of approximately 250,000 residents. A relatively new mental health care organization had recently moved into a new and ultra modern facility and was desiring to better understand its position with the local referral agents in the market. It was determined that four samples from groups determined to be potential local referral agents would be surveyed. Those groups included ministers/priests, public school counselors, medical doctors, business owners/leaders, and a sytematic random sample of general population households taken from the local phone directory.

A self-administered questionnaire was mailed to members of the various samples. A breakdown of the return rates is presented in Table 1. Counselors provided the best response rate followed by the

TABLE 1. Sample Design

Group	Question-naires Sent Out	Effective Size of Each Sample	Total Returns	Usable Returns	Effec-tive Percent Returned
	96	83	35	35	42%
School ce lors	50	50	38	38	76%
ians	267	264	66	61	23%
s ss	243	241	87	86	36%
tion	317	313	45	41	13%
	963	951	268	261	27%

clergy and business leaders. The response rates of physicians was above 20 percent, while the response rate from the general public was even lower after follow-up letters were sent out.

Questionnaire Development

To explore the local norm dimensions previously discussed in the literature review section, a series of 6-point Likert-scaled attitude statements were developed and pretested. The individual statements were then adjusted for clarity before being administered to the various samples. The revised series of Likert statements were directed towards a variety of attitude objects in Section I of the questionnaire. The attitude objects included issues of confidentiality, stigmas associated with mental health, self-improvement using mental health programs, who should pay for mental health care services, along with prevention and mental health education.

Section II of the questionnaire asked the respondents how likely they would be to discuss a personal mental health problem with each of 10 potential mental health referral agents. Finally, Section III of the questionnaire asked the respondents to what degree they felt it was important for a person to seek mental health care treatment if that person had 1 of 11 mental health problems. Each question was designed to focus on local norm differences across the various referral groups.

Data Analysis Procedures

The primary analysis technique employed in the study was discriminant analysis. Discriminant analysis is an application typically used to both explain and predict the effects that several metrically scaled predictor variables might have on a categorical dependent variable. The technique also provides the researcher with the ability to identify major dimensions, similar to factors, that differentiate among the categorical groups (Cooley and Lohnes, 1971). The SPSSX procedure (1986) was used for analysis purposes in this article. The stepwise sub-procedure based on the Wilk's lambda statistic was used to determine which independent predictor variables were retained to explain differences across the five potential referral subgroups that were sampled.

The procedure also provided mean and standard deviation statistics. Significance tests (paired F-tests) were used to indicate where significant differences existed between pairs of referral groups.

RESULTS

Attitude Differences by Subgroups

The discriminant analysis procedure resulted in 25 attitude variables being retained in the final solution (see Table 2). The F statistics between every pair of referral groups were all significant at the .05 level, thus indicating that the attitude variables were useful in distinguishing between the targeted referral groups. Four canonical discriminant functions were derived from the analysis (see Table 3). Three of the functions were significant at the .05 level reproducing over 88 percent of the variance from the attitude variables.

An examination of the discriminating factors can be useful in explaining the attitude characteristic differences of the five referral agent groups. Table 4 presents the correlations of those attitude statements with the four canonical functions. The nature of these factors suggests a closer look as to how each factor relates to referral groups' attitude characteristics toward mental health issues. The maximum loading of each variable indicates the strength of association between the individual attitude statement and the canonical discriminant function.

Individual's responsibility for mental health costs. The first discriminant function was named "Individual responsibility for mental health costs" since it correlates highly with the statement "I would be willing to pay for mental health services if I needed them," and negatively with the statement that insurance should pay for mental health costs. The function was responsible for explaining over 40 percent of the variation in the data. It appears that the first discriminant function simply reflects where the individual referral group stands on the individual being responsible for his or her own expenses for personal mental health care treatment, as opposed to the treatment being paid for by insurance or other sources (i.e., the government, employer, etc.).

Personal mental health/self improvement. The second discriminant function was closely correlated with three statements associated with a willingness towards, and a concern for, improving one's personal effectiveness characteristics and the limiting of potential mental health problems. This function explained 33.56 percent of the variation and as such has been given the label of "personal self-improvement."

Sources of mental health care resources. The third significant function explained 14.82 percent of the variation in the data. This function is strongly correlated positively with the belief that mental health care centers provide the best care for mental health problems and that it takes a strong person to seek help for a mental adjustment problem. The last statement again brings in the "stigma" concept as being an important consideration when treatment is being considered. The function is negatively correlated with the statement that prevention is an important part of a good mental health program.

Likelihood of having a problem and finding quality care. Although the final discriminant function was not statistically significant at the .05 level, it did explain the remaining 11.58 percent of the variation in the data. The function is strongly correlated with the statements that "Everyday people like you and me can experience temporary mental health problems" and other statements relating to the importance of confidentiality. The function was also negatively correlated with the statement that "Excellent health care is available in my community." This last statement would be quite useful in understanding which referral groups hold positive attitudes toward the existing treatment center and which referral groups will need to be targeted to improve negative image issues.

Relationship of Referral Groups to Attitude Dimensions

The discriminant factors are quite useful in understanding the differences among the various groups of respondents that were examined. These factors/constructs can help mental health care providers when trying to determine which groups hold attitudes which make them immediately useful as referral agents, as well as which groups will require more targeted marketing efforts. Table 5 presents the standardized factor/construct centroids (means) for

TABLE 2. Mental Health Care Attitude Means Across Five Referral Agent Groups

Attitude Variable	Clergy	Counselors
The term "mental health" means more than just treating people with mental disorders	5.08	5.67
Mental health care centers provide the best care for mental health problems.	3.44	3.37
I would consider attending seminars or classes which would help to improve my personal effectiveness.	4.52	5.17
I would be willing to pay for mental health services if I needed them.	5.00	5.53
Insurance should pay for an individual's mental health care services.	4.92	5.27
A person can be physically fit but not be mentally fit.	5.04	5.17
"Mental health" relates to normal, well-adjusted, people.	4.00	4.67
Most people, at some time or another, could use professional help with their mental health.	4.60	4.90

Physicians	Business People	General Population	Grand Mean	Sig * Level
4.70	5.05	4.93	5.50	.0000
3.34	4.00	3.83	3.64	.0027
3.81	4.43	3.93	4.33	.0000
5.21	5.36	4.93	5.24	.0014
4.19	4.36	4.53	4.56	.0000
5.36	5.30	5.57	5.30	.2777
4.64	3.97	3.73	4.21	.0124
3.96	4.48	4.73	4.47	.0013

TABLE 2 (continued)

Attitude Variable	Clergy	Counselors
I believe I would feel uneasy in a "mental health" building or office.	2.72	2.10
Excellent mental health care treatment is available in my community.	4.32	4.10
Everyday people, like you and me, can experience temporary mental health problems.	4.72	5.57
I would only go to a mental health care facility if I were sure that only my family would know about it.	2.88	3.17
Prevention is an important part of a good mental health program.	5.24	5.53
Family problems can often be related to mental health problems.	4.60	5.23
I would know where to go if I needed professional mental health care.	4.76	5.50
Mental Health issues are not well understood by the general public.	4.88	4.83

Physicians	Business People	General Population	Grand Mean	Sig * Level
2.98	2.93	2.87	2.78	.0129
4.19	4.74	4.13	4.36	.0116
5.13	4.98	5.00	5.07	.0126
3.34	2.93	2.90	3.06	.4436
4.79	4.90	4.63	4.97	.0008
4.87	4.97	4.73	4.90	.0968
4.89	4.84	4.33	4.87	.0016
4.57	4.79	5.03	4.79	.2218

TABLE 2 (continued)

Attitude Variable	Clergy	Counselors
Alcoholism is a major mental health problem in our community.	4.68	5.17
I have a positive feeling about mental fitness.	5.00	5.37
I feel that I understand the term "mental health."	4.80	5.40
Mental health problems can interfere with a person making a living.	5.16	5.80
I have a positive feeling about the term "mental health."	4.56	5.23
It takes a strong person to seek help for a mental adjustment problem.	3.88	4.00
The community should pay for an individual's mental health care services.	2.76	2.53
Americans do not spend enough money on preventing mental health problems.	4.64	4.83
I would not attend any classes or seminars which were held in a mental health facility.	2.12	1.70

*Wilk's Lambda (U-statistic) and univariate F-ratio with 4 and 188 degrees of freedom

Physicians	Business People	General Population	Grand Mean	Sig * Level
4.98	4.49	4.53	4.75	.0360
4.66	5.00	4.87	4.95	.0096
5.00	4.74	4.87	4.93	.0009
5.28	5.41	5.23	5.38	.0048
4.30	4.33	4.47	4.51	.0003
3.87	4.26	4.30	4.08	.2506
2.45	2.34	2.50	2.48	.6339
4.09	4.10	4.20	4.30	.0046
2.85	2.39	2.30	2.35	.0001

Table 3. Canonical Discriminant Functions of Mental Health Attitudes Across Five Sub-Populations.

Eigen Value	% of Variance Explained	Canonical Correlation	Wilks Lambda	Chi Square	Degrees of Freedom	Sig Level
			.267	234.1	100	0.
.649	40.03	.627	.440	145.5	72	0.
.544	33.56	.594	.679	68.6	46	0.
.240	14.82	.440	.842	30.5	22	0.
.188	11.58	.398				

each referral group on each of the previously described functions (i.e., constructs). The centroids for each group have been standardized to help in interpreting each group's position on the resulting functions.

Clergy. The clergy group was quite similar to the school counselor group and the general population sample group in that all of the groups were negative toward the idea of the individual being totally responsible for the cost of mental health care treatment. The clergy group was somewhat neutral regarding the use of mental health care center programs for self-improvement, but generally appeared to be supportive of the basic philosophies and services of mental health care centers. In short, this referral group may have some concerns about the local mental health center which need to be addressed.

Public school counselors. The public school counselor group was very knowledgeable and concerned about mental health issues. They strongly hold that the individual should not be entirely responsible for his or her mental health care treatment costs. As expected, this group is also extremely supportive of self-improvement programs offered by mental health care centers. This group is very supportive of mental health care centers in general, and appears to be strongly in favor of services to help prevent mental health problems. This group can be very important referral agents for the mental health care center.

Physicians. As expected, physicians were also very knowledgeable about mental health issues. Of all the groups examined, however, this group indicated the least amount of confidence in the care provided by mental health care centers. This may be related to physicians' overriding training to deal primarily with physiological issues. The physician group strongly feels that the individual should be responsible for his or her own mental health care costs. In general, the group is not supportive of mental health care centers nor the programs which they offer to the community. Whether the reason for this group's attitudes is a concern for a potential loss of patients, or a general mistrust of nonphysical ailments, clearly the physicians group represents a significant challenge for the marketer attempting to develop physicians as a referral group.

Business leaders. The business leader group appears to recognize

TABLE 4. Correlations Between Discriminant Functions/Factors and Agreement
with Mental Health Attitude Statements

Factor/Variables	Maximum Loading
Factor 1:	
--I would be willing to pay for mental health care services if I needed them.	.76
--Insurance should pay for an individual's mental health care services.	-.51
Factor 2:	
--I would consider attending seminars and classes which would help to improve my personal effectiveness.	.52
--A person can be physically fit but not mentally fit.	-.49
--Mental health problems can interfere with a person making a living.	.35
Factor 3:	
--Mental health care centers provide the best care for mental health problems.	.58
--Prevention is an important part of a good mental health program.	-.51
--It takes a strong person to seek help for a mental adjustment problem.	.43
Factor 4:	
--Everyday people like you and me can experience temporary mental health problems.	.58
--Excellent mental health care is available in my community.	.55
--I would only go to a mental health care facility if I were sure that only my family would know about it.	.53

the importance of mental health care centers as a significant community agency for providing mental health care treatment. This group is similar to the physicians group in that both strongly feel the individual should pay for his own mental health care. This finding is likely related to the basic business concern for maintaining low fixed operating costs, including taxes and insurance premiums. This group can best be approached by mental health care centers by arguing that positive mental health care programs and treatments can be cost effective for business in terms of lower workman's compensation claims, etc.

General population. As a group the general population sample is

Factor Level of Significance	Construct Name
.0000	Individual's Cost Responsibility
.0000	Personal Self Improvement
.0170	Sources of MH Help
.1076	Likelihood of any problems and quality care

less knowledgeable about mental health issues when compared to the other groups. This is not unexpected given the high education levels of the other groups. The general population sample does not feel that the individual should be entirely responsible for his or her mental health care costs. This group was not very interested in self-improvement and effectiveness courses that could be offered by mental health centers but they very strongly felt that mental health care centers provide the best care for mental health problems. Perhaps the former finding is related to the "stigma" concern previously discussed in the literature review. Another possibility is a true lack of interest or concern about mental health issues.

TABLE 5. Standardized Discriminant Function/Construct Centroids for Potential Referral Groups

Group	1	2	3	4	N	Percent of Sample
Clergy/ Priests	-.74	.20	-.68	-1.38	35	13.4%
Public School Counselor	-.86	1.53	-.51	.97	38	14.6%
Physicians	1.17	- .69	-.96	.95	61	23.3%
Business Leaders	1.00	.03	.94	-.50	86	33.0%
General Population	-.58	-1.07	1.21	-.05	41	15.7%

Discriminant function construct names:

1 = Individual's Cost Responsibility
2 = Personal Self Improvement
3 = Sources of MH Help
4 = Likelihood of mental health problem and quality of care

The differences of the various referral groups on the canonical discriminant functions illuminate a variety of useful attitude differences that mental health centers can use in developing strategies to cultivate referral agents. Other sources of useful information include differences in how referral groups view local problems and other mental health service providers.

Preferred Referral Agent Across Groups

The results of the question of how likely each respondent would be to contact different potential referral agents and care providers if the respondent personally had a mental health problem are presented in Table 6. As expected, clergy, counselors, and physicians were all highly inclined to contact someone in their respective professions. Spouses were also very likely to be contacted. This is not surprising since spouses are the most probable people for individuals to share their concerns and personal problems with.

Psychologists, private psychiatrists, physicians and friends had overall scores indicating higher likelihoods of being contacted about a personal problem than did the mental health center. This finding is quite interesting for the mental health facility operating in this market. It indicates that significant marketing effort will be required for the mental health care center to become an agent of choice for the potential referral agents.

Another interesting finding was that school counselors indicated significantly lower likelihoods of contacting a physician than any other source of help for personal problems. Somewhat related was the physicians group indicating the very lowest likelihood of contacting a mental health center. This presents a real problem since the other referral groups and the general population see the physician as a very likely place to go for mental health problem care.

Teachers and school counselors were not viewed as likely people to be contacted if personal mental health related problems were to occur. This low likelihood response may be due to the obvious lack of regular personal contact the other groups might have with teachers and counselors. As such it does suggest some interesting questions for the mental health center since teachers and counselors are

TABLE 6. Mean Scores as to How Likely Individuals from Five Sub-Populations Would Be to Contact a Specific Individual If They Each Had a Mental Fitness Problem

	Clergy	Couns-elors	Physi-ician	Bus-iness People	Gen-eral Popu-lation	Grand Mean	Sig. Level P
Friend	4.28	4.37	4.06	3.77	3.87	4.01	.49
Spouse	5.40	5.47	5.21	5.44	4.77	5.28	.10
Physician	4.96	3.97	4.89	4.85	5.07	4.77	.02
Mental Health Center	4.20	4.37	3.23	3.95	4.07	3.89	.02
Minister/ Priest	5.32	3.30	3.28	3.51	3.13	3.60	.00
Behavioral Medicine Clinic	3.28	2.80	2.62	2.85	2.73	2.82	.44
Teacher	2.36	2.37	1.98	1.93	1.87	2.06	.37
School Counselor	2.32	4.03	1.87	2.08	1.90	2.34	.00
Private Psychia-trists	3.84	4.30	4.87	4.11	4.20	4.31	.06
Psychol-ogist	4.20	5.00	4.55	4.48	3.80	4.44	.02

```
1= very unlikely          4= slightly likely
2= somewhat likely        5= somewhat likely
3= slightly unlikely      6= very likely
```

typically supportive of the efforts and programs found in mental health care centers.

It is equally obvious from this analysis that significant differences do exist regarding the way potential referral agents view the sources of help for mental care problems in the community. Such insights can be extremely helpful to local mental health care facilities in the development of effective local marketing plans.

Mental Health Problem Importance by Group

A series of mental health problems were presented to the respondents to be ranked in importance by level of need to seek mental health care. The results of this section of the questionnaire are presented in Table 7.

With the exception of the problems of "forgetfulness," "schizophrenia," "child abuse or incest," and "marital problems/divorce," significant differences do exist across the referral groups examined. Of the 4 problems discussed above, only "forgetfulness" was not considered to be of extremely high importance to all of the respondent groups.

Differences between the groups on the importance of the various mental health problems include the clergy and school counselors groups placing relatively higher importance on the problems related to potentially disruptive family issues such as alcoholism, rape, and fears. Physicians, however, placed significantly lower importance on these same issues. Another interesting contrast was the counselors group placing strong importance on depression, "life adjustment" problems, and stress when compared to the other groups. The 3 problems are the types of situations that counselors are likely to regularly face in their daily contacts with students. Physicians gave these same problems noticeably less importance. Perhaps physicians should be a strong target for contact from mental health care professionals to make them more aware of problems other than those of the physical nature.

DISCUSSION

With the increase in competition among mental health professionals for referrals, an increased concern for local norms and related issues appears to be a defensible approach for identifying and cultivating local referrals. Advertising and other marketing tools are likely to be more effective when properly mixed to create an overall marketing strategy based on solid information about the local market. The methodology presented in this article demonstrates how such information can be gathered and interpreted to be included in such a strategy.

TABLE 7. How Important Is It for People to Seek Mental Health Care for Eleven Problems
Mean Scores Across Five Respondent Groups

Problem	Clergy	Coun-selors	Phys-icians	Bus-iness People	Gen-eral Popul-ation	Grand Mean	Sig Level
Forgetfull-ness	2.20	2.37	2.36	2.33	2.17	2.30	.89
Rape	4.88	4.90	4.55	4.82	4.80	4.77	.01
Inability to get al-ong with friends & co-workers	4.28	4.40	3.94	4.16	4.00	4.13	.04
Alcohol	4.76	4.80	4.38	4.41	4.50	4.52	.04
Stress	3.80	4.10	3.45	3.75	3.83	3.75	.01
Depression	4.08	4.70	4.26	4.30	4.27	4.32	.01
Fears	3.72	4.13	3.43	3.72	3.67	3.70	.00
Life Adjustments	3.44	3.97	3.28	3.36	3.40	3.45	.00
Schizo-phrenia	4.64	4.93	4.74	4.67	4.63	4.72	.18
Child Abuse or Incest	4.96	5.00	4.89	4.93	5.00	4.95	.17
Marital Prb/Divorce	4.20	4.30	3.98	4.02	4.07	4.08	.37

1= not important
2= below average importance
3= average importance
4= above average importance
5= most important

Using the data gathered in the present study several possible strategies are suggested. First, the mental health center staff must recognize that no matter how good or professional they perceive themselves as being, the general population gave them a very average rating at best. The highest rating for mental health care centers came from the counselor and clergy groups. Based upon these findings, the mental health care center cannot view their present position as overly positive.

Perhaps the first step that should be taken by the mental health care center would be to determine the specific attributes used in judging mental health care providers. Using these characteristics as the basis for a consumer study, the mental health care center could determine specifically how and why different groups feel as they do. Perceptions could be weighed against actual characteristics to determine if the consumer was correct in their perceptions. Advertising, which might include direct mail, television, radio, or even outdoor signs could be used to target specific messages to specific markets. For example, the data reported in this study shows that school counselors presently hold mental health care centers in relatively high regard. Direct mail material sent to these counselors detailing the types of programs provided for youth by the mental health center would most likely be well received. More direct contact (personal selling) with physicians detailing the professional credentials of the mental health center staff may be the most effective method of changing the very low score (3.23) given by physicians in this study. The 4.77 grand mean given to physicians make them an important, if not vital, gatekeeper. While direct mail is a possibility, it seems unlikely that any other method of reaching physicians would be as effective as direct contact.

It is also possible that while psychiatrists and psychologists are direct competitors to mental heath centers, this may be a source of referral for the lower socio-economic consumer who cannot afford to pay a private providers fee. Again a direct contact with these individuals seems to be the most appropriate method for outlining the mental health care center's programs and capabilities.

In summary, each market must be viewed in terms of its perceptions and needs. Only after local norms are understood can effective targeting strategies be determined for reaching each referral group market.

REFERENCES

Ahmed, S. M. S. and Viswanathan, P. (1984), "Factor Analytical Study of Nunnally's Scale of Popular Concepts of Mental Health," *Psychological Reports*, 54, 455-461.

Cooley, William W., and Lohnes, Paul R. (1971), *Multivariate Data Analysis*, John Wiley & Sons, Inc., New York, 223-227.

Cox, G., Costanzo, P., and Cole, J. (1976), "A Survey Instrument for the Assessment of Popular Conceptions of Mental Health," *Journal of Consulting and Clinical Psychology*, 44, 6.

DeMello, Steven (1983-1984), "Market Planning for Mental Health: A 'Target Group' Based Approach," *Health Marketing Quarterly*, (Winter-Spring), 1, 13-17.

Farina, A., Fisher, J., Getter, H., and Fischer, E., (1978), "Some Consequences of Changing People's Views Regarding the Nature of Mental Health," *Journal of Abnormal Psychology*, 87, 2, 272-279.

Kohler, Marsha S. and Corrigan, John D. (1983-1984), "Public Attitudes Toward Community Mental Health: Services, Funding, and Voter Behavior," *Health Marketing Quarterly*, (Winter-Spring), 1, 39-56.

Morrison, J., Maorazo-Peterson, R., Simons, P., and Gold, B., (1977), "Attitudes Toward Mental Illness: A Conflict Between Students and Professionals," *Psychological Reports*, 41, 1013-1014.

Olmsted, D. and Durham, K. (1976), "Stability of Mental Health Attitudes: A Semantic Differential Study," *Journal of Health and Social Behavior*, (March), 17, 35-44.

Page, Stewart and Page, Susan (1974), "What is Psychiatric Stigma?", *Psychological Reports*, 34, 630.

Piner, Kelly and Kahle, Lynn (1984), "Adapting to Stigmatizing Labels of Mental Illness: Foregone But Not Forgotten," *Journal of Personality and Social Psychology*, 47, 4, 805-811.

Time (1986), "Polling for Mental Health," (October 15), 80.

SPSSX Users Guide, 2nd ed., SPSS Inc., Chicago, 1986, 688-712.

Stensrud, R. and Stensrud, K. (1980), "Attitudes Toward Successful Individuals With and Without Histories of Psychiatric Hospitalization," *Psychological Reports*, 47, 495-498.

Evolutionary Changes in the Marketing of Mental Health Products to Government, Business and Industry

James W. Busbin

SUMMARY. The U.S. mental health industry is growing, with government, business and industrial organizations playing an increasingly important role. Organizations have accepted the responsibility of employee stress management and incorporated it into existing employee wellness programs. Since stress is an artifact of mental health, it may serve as a link through which organizations eventually assume a central role in employee mental health management. With this will come major changes in the U.S. mental health market. Providers of mental health products could benefit strategically by evaluating these evolutionary changes.

INTRODUCTION

The mental health industry in America is large and growing, and important evolutionary changes are taking place concomitant with this growth. Over the next decade the parties involved in the production, distribution and consumption of mental health products and services will likely be redefining their form, functions and roles within the mental health industry. Responding to these evolutionary changes in the mental health market is particularly important for the providers of mental health products. Providers could suffer business

James W. Busbin, PhD, is Associate Professor of Marketing at Western Carolina University in Cullowhee, NC.

loss should they not stay abreast of shifts in demand, in terms of both product types and customer base.

Adapting to market changes has become relevant for government supported, nonprofit mental health providers as well. For example, the Community Mental Health Center (CMHC) system experienced a decline in government funding when the Omnibus Budget Reconciliation Act of 1981 repealed the legislation authorizing CMHCs and consolidated all federal funds for mental health and substance abuse into a single block grant providing 21% less support (Kline and Self, 1990). With lessened government support, Community Mental Health Centers are being forced to diversify and seek business in alternative markets, particularly the private sector.

In the early part of this century the mental health industry was rather simple and well structured. Only individuals who were chronically mentally ill became subjects of treatment or institutionalization — persons suffering moderate mental illness were without recourse and typically were dealt with by family, community or church. The individuals and organizations providing products and services were also straightforward; psychiatrists were the treatment agent, and government-supported hospitals and asylums were the functional institutions.

The simplistic structure which prevailed for decades began to undergo changes in the 1960s and 1970s. The U.S. Government instituted Medicare and Medicaid systems and hospitals were deregulated; this introduced the government as a third party payer while hospitals responded to deregulation with rapid expansions of facilities and services. Also, both private and public specialty mental health centers (e.g., private, specialty treatment centers and Community Mental Health Centers) emerged in response to the demand for counseling and the treatment of less chronic psychological conditions. When taken together, these and other developments have resulted in a mental health industry in a state of flux — roles are shifting and participants are redefining their form and function. When a settling-down eventually occurs, the producers, distributors and consumers of mental health products may well find themselves serving in capacities significantly different from previous years.

This article explores one path which this evolution in the mental health industry may plausibly follow — that U.S. employer organizations could emerge as the dominant party in the mental health marketplace. Employer organizations are playing an increasingly important and influential role in the lifestyle and health of their employees. Recently, this has been accomplished through the widespread adoption of employee wellness programs (Busbin, 1990).

Although employee wellness programs had humble beginnings, they have evolved into increasingly comprehensive programs for overall employee health maintenance. One remaining domain for wellness program expansion is mental health, and pretenses for absorbing this employee health category are being made through employee stress management. The further pursuit of stress management will eventually lead companies to accept employee mental health as an integral part of employee health maintenance.

Should these changes proceed, U.S. organizations will become America's largest, and most centralized, consumer of mental health products and services. Beyond being a mainstay consumer of mental health products, organizations may also function as "clearing houses" for the mental health market by centralizing referral activities and record keeping. The prospects of such developments have important ramifications for producers of mental health products; not only will the customer base change, but also the overall character of the mental health market. While these changes may precipitate an increase in the overall demand for mental health products, selling to centralized, cost-conscience organizations as consumers is quite different from selling to the present fragmented and disorganized market.

Employee wellness programs become relevant when considering employer organizations as consumers of mental health products. Where once organizations purchased health services on an as-needed basis, a large proportion of government, business and industrial organizations have now integrated all employee health-related matters into an employee wellness framework. Larger organizations often have highly organized wellness programs complete with dedicated facilities and on-site nurses, physicians and professional staff (Busbin, 1990). To consider U.S. organizations as prospective consumers of mental health products, one must consider the employee wellness structure through which the products would be purchased.

A BRIEF HISTORY OF EMPLOYEE WELLNESS

Employee wellness has its origins in worker safety standards founded during America's industrial expansion era in the early 1900s. From this point, and as industries became more mechanized, safety education became necessary. Worker illness was also a problem during these times with epidemics not uncommon. Thus, the U.S. Federal Government became the first major practitioner of health education by dispensing information on communicable diseases and other health-related causes of employee absenteeism.

In the decades of the 1930s, 1940s and 1950s employee assistance programs and health screening services emerged. Employee assistance programs in this period focused largely on alcoholism while health screening sought early detection of communicable diseases. It was also during this era that labor unions began to promote employee health support as a company-provided employee fringe benefit.

The 1970s ushered in a new era in employee health; health *promotion* was introduced. The important difference here is that health promotion represented a shift from strictly corrective medicine (resolving health problems after they occur) to preventative medicine, or striving to prevent health problems from occurring in the first place. Two main phenomena influenced the introduction and growth of a preventative approach to employee health: (1) Advances in medical knowledge about good health, coupled with health-related employee lifestyle interests (jogging, etc.), resulted in a higher level of employee concern about good health and company health care support, and (2) the escalating costs of providing employee health care coverage forced companies to explore alternative cost control remedies, preventative medicine being among them.

Employee health care cost control appears to be the primary impetus for organizations to develop employee wellness programs. Of course, a number of other reasons for instituting employee wellness programs are commonly cited, for example, humanitarian concern for worker well being, personal interest in fitness by company executives, improved worker productivity, enhanced retention of valuable employees, and so forth. However, American corporations paid more than $87 million in health care premiums in 1985 — an amount greater than the total paid to stockholders that year (Wagel, 1989). In 1990, premiums likely will total $640 million, or roughly 11% of the Gross National Product (Katzman and Smith, 1989). Further, Welling (1990) observes that at its current rate of growth, better than two times the rate of the consumer price index, health care threatens to claim a staggering one out of every five dollars the economy produces by the year 2000. In summary, reducing employee health care costs has become an organizational priority, and employee wellness programs are thought to be one means of doing this.

U.S. organizations are optimistic that employee wellness programs will more than pay for themselves in the long run by reducing employees' needs for corrective health services; the notion here is that an ounce of prevention is worth a pound of cure. Major benefits which organizations hope to receive from employee wellness programs include: (a) reduction of employee benefit costs associated with health and workman's compensation, (b) reduction of the costs of replacing valued workers lost to injury or illness, (c) positive employee response in expressing concern for worker well being, (e) enhanced productivity of retained employees, and (d) increased employee retention by providing an additional benefit (Howard and Mikalachki, 1979; Pyle, 1979; Cox, 1982; Shepard and Pearlman, 1985; *Dun's*, 1985, 1986; Patterson, 1986; Eriksen, 1988; *Public Health Reports*, 1987; Smith, 1987; and Chen, 1988).

THE TRANSITION OF EMPLOYEE WELLNESS TOWARD MENTAL HEALTH SERVICES

Employee wellness programs have evolved through a number of stages since their origins in the early 1900s and formalization in the 1970s. Essentially, the pattern of development of employee wellness programs has been a logical one; the first health concerns to be addressed were obvious ones having immediate and observable impact (e.g., on-the-job injury and communicable diseases). Then, as each health issue was resolved, wellness programs would move progressively along to the next in line. Correspondingly, each progressive health issue became more long-term in scope and more comprehensive in nature.

STAGE 1: Occupational Safety — Beginning during the American industrial revolution, safe employee working conditions became the first cause championed by employee labor unions. The U.S. government came to play an active role in employee safety as well through the Labor Department and the eventual establishment of the Occupational Safety and Health Administration (OSHA). Today, the elimination of on-the-job hazards and provisions for worker safety are standard business practice.

STAGE 2: Substance Abuse and Employee Assistance Programs — Alcoholism among employees has plagued employers throughout history, with U.S. organizations initially adopting policies of toleration, accommodation or termination. Few companies aspired to help correct the situation, with lack of knowledge on how to go about doing so also prevailing. Then in the 1950s American organizations began to formally address employee alcoholism by establishing occupational alcoholism programs (OAPs). Stories of successful treatment programs began to stimulate widespread interest among U.S. organizations and OAPs began to spread (Franco, 1957). By the early 1960s about 100 occupational alcoholism programs existed nationwide, but an explosion of growth throughout the 1970s and 1980s resulted in thousands of such programs being established (Kurtz, Googins and Howard, 1984).

Today, occupational alcoholism programs have evolved into employee assistance programs (EAPs) with broader ranges of concern. Organizational EAPs typically provide employee support regarding substance abuse and psychological problems as well as alcoholism.

STAGE 3: Employee Health Screening — Screening for health problems began with efforts to detect communicable diseases in the early 1900s. However, health screening today has assumed a more sophisticated, preventative role. Employees may be regularly checked for such conditions and health risk factors as high blood pressure, glaucoma, diabetes, and so forth. A primary goal of employee health screening is early detection thus enhancing treatment and cure, or avoiding a potential health problem altogether.

STAGE 4: Exercise and Physical Fitness — Organizational concern with employee physical fitness perhaps marked the beginning of the transition toward a preventative approach to employee health problems. Advances in the medical understanding of health and pathology exposed exercise to be a basic ingredient in good health. Also, employee acceptance of the exercise/good health link was augmented by newfound recreational fitness activities (e.g., jogging, racket ball, etc.). Consequently, organizations found that employees would readily accept exercise and fitness components of employee wellness programs.

STAGE 5: Employee Health Education — Education has long been a part of company wellness activities, but with the recent adoption of a preventative philosophy has expanded to become a mainstay of employee wellness programs. Providing wellness education programs to government, business and industry is now a multimillion dollar market for health product providers. The diverse topics to be found in wellness education include prenatal child care, personal nutrition and meal planning, stress management, how to stop smoking, heart attack prevention, first aid and CPR, personal breast examination for early cancer detection, and numerous others.

STAGE 6: Nutritional Counseling and Diet Control — For decades select organizations have offered on-premises dining for employees. As knowledge relating diet to health accumulated, organizations began to employ the company dining hall in dispensing information and conforming behavior. Meal planners and nutritional counselors became commonplace by the 1980s. Today, nutritional education and/or on-premises meal planning is an integral part of the vast majority of wellness programs.

STAGE 7: Rehabilitation — In earlier years, rehabilitation was tantamount to "recovery." When workers were lost to illness or injury organizations were content to allow healing to proceed at its own pace. Since then, medical advances have shown that active rehabilitation programs can accelerate recovery rates thus returning workers back to the job much sooner. For government, business and industry, shorter recovery periods convert to millions of dollars saved in medical costs and lost employee productivity (*National Safety News*, 1984). Thus, professionally developed rehabilitation programs have become an active part of employers' health care provisions.

STAGE 8: Stress Management — Stress became a common "buzzword" in the 1970s and 1980s. The popular press was replete with stress management techniques and entrepreneurs staged stress management seminars. Unlike other transient topics in business, however, the emerging medical implications of stress solidified it as a major concern both in business practice and medical research. Today, the effects of job-related stress on employees is being studied closely. Furthermore, a large proportion of organizations formally address the problem of employee stress through such actions as educational seminars and environmental control.

STAGE 9: Holistic Management — This stage is set in the future several decades from now. As the evolution continues organizations may come to realize the central role they play in the lives of their employees and assume a position of influence and control. Further medical advances would provide well-defined cause and effect relationships between employee health and the environmental influences. Such circumstances would be conducive for organizations to practice a holistic approach to employee health management; employee health would be viewed as an agent of the environment as a whole, with the work environment being paramount.

STRESS MANAGEMENT AS A LINK
TO MENTAL HEALTH PRODUCTS

The array of employee health services itemized in the previous section's nine stages represent an evolutionary spectrum of development. At the earliest extreme employers were concerned only with first aid and accident prevention. At the opposite, future extreme is found a very broad regard for employee health as it functions within a total realm of environmental influence. Presently, U.S. organizations find themselves somewhere in between, with positions varying from organization to organization. Generally, progressive organizations have evolved up to the point of recognizing stress as a health factor, with most attempting some form of counteractive measures (e.g., soothing color schemes, sound insulation, "work break" schedules, stress management classes, etc.). Should organizations continue to evolve relative to their interpretations of employee health, and there appears no reason why they should not, then it is only a matter of time before employee mental health becomes formally included in the employee health agenda.

Medical research plays an influential role in organizations' practice of employee wellness, and evidence which links stress to mental illness continues to mount. For example, Kahn and Quinn linked stress to coronary heart disease and mental illness in experimental settings (1970) and Margolis, Kroes and Quinn confirmed the same linkage in work place settings (1974). Psychosocial stress can increase susceptibility to infectious disease as well as inhibit recovery from disease; the immune system is modulated by the brain, which is affected by stress, thus, psychosocial stress can disrupt the immune system rendering people more vulnerable to physical, chemical or biological maladies (1980). Further, in 1989 Lahey reported from the *American Journal of Health Promotion* that "Both basic and clinical experimental research have determined stress to be a major factor in a wide range of conditions including hypertension, cardiovascular disease, gastrointestinal disorders, tension and vascular headaches, low back pain and decreased immunological functioning with its implications for susceptibility to disorders ranging from colds and flu to cancer and AIDS" (p. 53). The means by which stress serves as a linkage to mental and physical health is well articulated by Schwartz:

> We are witnessing today a major change in our conception of
> health and illness. In the past, psychological and biological
> models of health and illness were couched in separate languages and practiced as separate disciplines — now these separations are being broken down. . . . The concept of stress and

its implications for health and illness is a key factor bringing
these disparate disciplines together. (1980, p. 100)

Figure 1, "Relationship of Stress to Mental Illness," depicts the
manner in which stress originates and relates to other important
aspects of behavior, physical health, and importantly, to mental
illness.

Figure 1 dichotomizes the origins of stress into on-the-job
sources and away-from-the-job sources. On-the-job sources have
been categorized by various authors into five main categories; factors intrinsic to job, role in organization, career development, relationships at work, and organizational structure and climate (Cooper

FIGURE 1

Relationship of Stress to Mental Illness

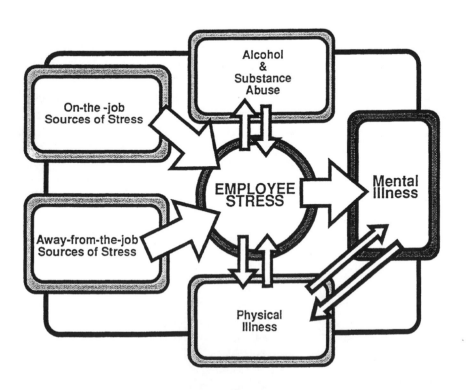

and Marshall, 1976; Magnuson, 1990). While attention has been focused on job-related stress for relatively few years, much progress in its understanding has occurred.

Away-from-the-job sources of stress have received less organized study than has job-related stress, with family problems, life crises, and financial difficulties receiving the most attention. The greatest shortcoming in the study of stress concerns understanding the relationships between on-the-job and away-from-the-job sources of stress. In order for substantial advances to occur in stress management, employees' environmental stress as a whole will need to be better understood.

Figure 1 indicates two-way relationships between employee stress and alcohol and substance abuse, and stress and physical illness. As cited in previous research, considerable evidence suggests these relationships exist. For example, Ivancevich and Matteson note that the chronic, stress-related diseases of adulthood (e.g., coronary heart disease, stroke, hypertension, cancer, emphysema, diabetes, cirrhosis, and suicide) have now become the leading causes of death (1980). Also, it is generally accepted that substance abuse and alcoholism are often merely symptoms of stress-related psychological problems as opposed to root source problems themselves.

The final extension of Figure 1 links employee stress to mental illness. The assumption here is of advanced stress overload, to the extent that the employee develops clinically measurable neurosis such as depression, phobias, severe anxiety, nervous breakdowns, or other such handicapping mental problems.

THE MULTIPLE OUTCOMES
OF EMPLOYEE STRESS OVERLOAD

Stress overload became a popular research subject in the 1970s, and remains a topic of interest up to the present. The effects of stress have been studied by an array of authorities from medical scientists to organizational behavior specialists. As a result, much has been learned about the relationship of stress to various outcomes. Figure 2, "Outcomes of Employee Stress Overload," itemizes a number of stress-related outcomes by category. The medical and organizational behavior literature is replete with the kind of

FIGURE 2

Outcomes of Employee Stress Overload

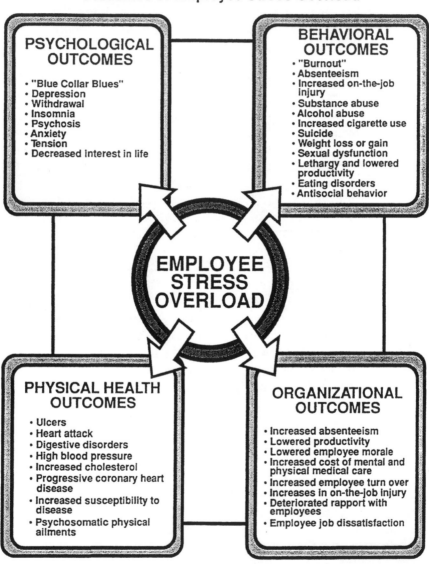

findings represented in Figure 2. Rather than delve into an extensive review of this literature, Figure 2 simply presents a sampling of outcomes and organizes them into respective categories. From this, further understanding can be gained about the central role which stress appears to play in mental and physical health and job performance.

GOVERNMENT, BUSINESS AND INDUSTRY AS CONSUMERS OF MENTAL HEALTH PRODUCTS

The marketing delivery system for mental health products in the United States has been somewhat unstructured. This, when combined with the elusive nature of mental problems, the stigma of treatment, and the general level of societal misunderstandings, results in an ambiguous product category. Ambiguity in a marketing system can prove to be frustrating to both product providers and consumers in the system. Providers experience difficulty in accessing and communicating with consumers, and consumers are stymied in understanding product need and seeking appropriate product providers.

The disparate nature of the mental health delivery system may potentially be resolved as the role of government, business and industry in the mental health industry evolves over the next decade; employer organizations may begin to function as "central clearing houses" or "channel captains" for the mental health industry. There are a number of reasons why employer organizations may begin to assume a more centralized role in mental health delivery systems. These variables can be categorized into the following main groups:

Legal Obligations

Several court cases have set a precedent holding employers responsible for mental health problems which employees could relate to job working conditions. For example, a Colorado fireman died from "a pre-existing heart problem aggravated by job-related mental stress." The Colorado Supreme Court reversed the findings of a workman's compensation referee and held the employer responsible for the fireman's death. The Colorado high court said that stress is a disease in its own right and can be implicated in many other diseases and disabilities (Lahey, 1989). In another instance, an executive employee sued his employer claiming that his work caused him psychological ailments, physiological ailments, and finally, a heart attack. The man won his case and the company was ordered to pay him a cash settlement (Ivancevich and Matteson, 1980). Thus, U.S. organizations may have little discretion in whether or not to assume some degree of responsibility for the mental health of their employees — the assumption may need to be made out of defensive necessity.

Exposure to Employees in a Structured Environment and Incentive to Confront Mental Health Problems

Mental health problems are more troublesome to detect, identify and treat than are physical health problems. This is true for two reasons: (1) mental health problems manifest themselves in a variety of ways and often do not produce pronounced, easy-to-recognize symptoms until an advanced stage (i.e., a "breakdown" of some kind), and (2) due to the stigma attached to mental illness, persons involved with an afflicted individual often choose to avoid the reality of the problem (i.e., hope it will go away unaided, mask the symptoms with medication, strive to find physical problems to blame for the condition, etc.). Employer organizations are in a unique position to redress both of these barriers to effective resolution of mental health problems. First, employers have day-to-day exposure to employees in a structured setting. Early detection of a mental health problem requires a comparison of present behavior against a longer-term "track record." Thus, job performance serves as an ideal barometer of mental stability. Indeed, co-workers often report psychological problems long before they would have been noticed in a family setting. Second, employers have an incentive to confront employee psychological problems instead of "sidestepping" them. Beyond the legal implications of deferred treatment, allowing a problem to persist costs an organization money through lowered productivity, absenteeism and so forth.

Heightened Understanding of Employee Mental Problems

In years past, the understanding of mental health problems, especially of the less chronic variety, was rudimentary. Government, business and industry did little regarding employee mental health for it was an enigma. Today, the understanding of mental health is greatly advanced. Linkages among stress, the work environment and psychological and physical maladies are more clear. Employers are no longer handicapped by a general lack of understanding of employee mental health. Moreover, research has distinctively linked work environment to stress, stress to mental health, and mental health to physical health. Employers have been forced to acknowledge the evident role which the work environment plays in the overall mental condition of employees.

Economic Incentives

The basic premise underlying the rapid adoption of employee wellness programs is an economic one; healthy employees require less medical care, and the costs of employee wellness programs are thus more than offset by health care cost savings. The organization enjoys happier, more productive employees while simultaneously saving on costly health insurance premiums. Employee mental health problems have received less attention in employee wellness than other, more obtrusive health concerns, but this may change as the understanding of the prevalence and impact of employee psychological conditions continues to advance. For example, early studies found that up to 30% of workers in manufacturing settings suffered from some form of neurosis in a six-month time frame (Aldridge, 1970). Further, in 1969 the Department of Health and Social Security in Great Britain reported that 22.8 million work days that year were lost to "mental, psychoneurotic and personality disorders, nervousness, and headache." This placed mental illness in second place in terms of days lost, behind bronchitis, but ahead of heart disease (Aldridge, 1970). Lastly, Schwartz reported that among participants in an Emotional Health Program at Equitable Life Assurance Corporation 58% of the men and 36% of the women cited job-related stress factors as contributing to their problems (1980).

Lack of Alternative Means of Detection and Treatment

One could argue that U.S. organizations may assume a central role in the mental health delivery system by default; there may be no other logical alternative. The employment environment provides the exposure and work standards necessary for early detection. Also, an incentive to address and correct the problem exists on both the part of the employer and employee; the employer saves money while retaining valuable employees and employees receive the outside help necessary to relieve themselves of mental problems while retaining their job.

CONCLUSION

This article reviews the evolutionary changes which are occurring in the American mental health care market. A particular focus has been on organizational employee wellness programs and the progressive link through stress management which may lead employer organizations toward centralized involvement with the mental health industry. Should the evolution of employee wellness programs continue on as it has for the past twenty years, then inclusion of employee mental health as an organizational responsibility is only a matter of time. Indeed, the transition toward assuming greater responsibility for employee mental health appears to be well underway given the increasing mental health service utilization by employees, for example, Lawless explains that:

> Many employers have recently seen a rapid rise in the cost of their mental health benefits, far beyond that of their traditional medical care costs. . . . The rate of utilization among employers for all mental health services has more than doubled in the past few years. According to Blue Cross and Blue Shield studies, many employers have seen a rapid increase in their budg-

etary allocation for mental health services, from 15% in the mid 1980s to as high as 30% by 1988. This trend is expected to continue, with an anticipated rise to 40% of an employer's total health care costs going to psychiatric and substance abuse benefits by the early 1990s. (1990, p. 6)

As implied by these figures, the monetary costs of poor employee mental health can be compelling. For example, the United States Clearing House for Mental Health information reports that U.S. industry suffers a $17 billion annual decrease in productivity because of stress-induced mental dysfunctions (Ivancevich and Matteson, 1980). Economic repercussions of this severity can exert considerable pressure for change on organizations. And in response employer organizations in the United States appear to be changing toward becoming preeminent players in the mental health delivery system. Organizations will be playing multiple roles in this capacity. They will be both primary consumers for employee mental health services, especially for less chronic conditions such as stress management, and also serve in referral or "clearing house" capacities. This prospective evolutionary change in the mental health care market will have far-reaching effects on all of its participants. Producers of mental health products and services will be particularly affected. Product providers may encounter changes regarding their:

Customer Base – Large, employer organizations could come to dominate the consumption market for mental health products and services.

Product and Service Selection – Employer organizations may play an active role in specifying products and services, monitoring quality, seeking evaluation of results, and so forth.

Nature and Method of Payment – Organizations often maintain strict accountability of expenses and long payment periods. The personnel responsible for negotiating payment may be far removed from the personnel originally procuring the services.

Sales Methods – Selling mental health products and services to employer organizations, for third-party consumption, may be quite different from selling to the smaller and more diverse client base which many mental health companies serve today. Employer organizations may employ "proposals" or "submitting bids" approaches to vendor acquisition.

Distribution System — If the customer base changes, then the distribution methods to service those customers will also change. Providers of mental health products and services may find themselves further removed from customers, or be required to deliver services to diverse and changing locations (e.g., divisions of a company with separate locations).

Communications systems — Achieving effective communication with large organizations is generally more difficult than with smaller ones. Identifying and reaching organizational decision makers could be challenging, and frustrating.

Nature of the Ultimate Consumer — The principle behind why patients appear for treatment may shift with organizational sponsorship. In some instances organizations may coerce employees to submit to treatment under the threat of termination. Thus, subtle accommodations in treatment methods may be required.

In summary, it appears plausible that U.S. employer organizations may evolve into dominating the mental health marketplace in America. This eventuality could provide both opportunities and pitfalls for other participants in the mental health market. Opportunities await those willing to monitor the evolutionary changes in the mental health market and strategically plan for their role within it. Pitfalls may await those who wait until change is forced upon them by an unyielding market. At the present, both options are available.

REFERENCES

Aldridge, J.F.L. (1970), "Emotional Illness and the Working Environment," *Ergonomics*, Vol. 13, No. 5, 613-621.

Busbin, James W. (1990), "Market Evolutions in Health Care and the Emergence of Employee Wellness as a New Product Category," *Health Marketing Quarterly,* Vol. 7, Nos. 3/4, 7-22.

Chen, M.S. Jr. (1988), "Wellness in the Workplace: Beyond the Point of No Return," *Health Values,* 12,1 (January/February): 16-22.

Cooper, Cary L. and Judi Marshall (1976), "Occupational Sources of Stress: A Review of the Literature Relating to Coronary Heat Disease and Mental Ill Health," *Journal of Occupational Health*, 1976, No. 49, 11-28.

Cox, M.H. (1982), "Corporate Investment in Human Resources: A New Twist," *Canadian Business Review*, 9 (Spring): 9-14.

Dun's-Business Month (1985), "Executive Fitness," 126 (December): 41-42.

_____(1986), "Executive Health Update '86," 128 (July): 50-54.

Eriksen, M.P. (1988), "The Role of Cancer Prevention in Workplace Health Promotion," *Health Values*, 12,2 (March/April): 18-23.

Franco, S.C. (1957), "Problem Drinking in Industry: Review of a Company Program," *Ind. Med. Surg.*, 26:221-228.

Howard, J. and Mikalachki, A. (1979), "Fitness and Employee Productivity," *Canadian Journal of Applied Sport Sciences*, Vol. 4, No. 3, 191-8.

Ivancevich, J.M. and Matteson, M.T. (1980), "Optimizing Human Resources: A Case for Preventive Health and Stress Management," *Organizational Dynamics*, (Autumn): 5-25.

Kahn, R.L. and Quinn, R.P. (1970), "Role Stress," *Mental Health and Work Organization*, 50-115.

Katzman, M.S. and Smith, K.J. (1989), "Occupational Health-Promotion Programs: Evaluation Efforts and Measured Cost Savings," *Health Values*, 13,2 (March/April): 3-10.

Kline, Teri and Donald R. Self (1990), "Future Directions for Marketing Community Mental Health Centers: The Referral System Perspective," *Journal of Marketing for Mental Health*, Vol 2, Number 2, 61-85.

Kurtz, N.R., Googins, B., & Howard, W.C. (1984), "Measuring the Success of Occupational Alcoholism Programs," *Journal of Studies in Alcohol*, Vol. 45, No. 1, 33-4.

Lahey, J. (1989), "Stress," *Safety and Health*, 139(6), 53-5.

Lawless, G.D. (1990), "Cost Containment Through Outpatient Substance Abuse Services," *Employee Benefits Journal*, (March): 6-10.

Magnusonl, John (1990), "Stress Management," *Journal of Property Management*, May/June, 24-27.

Margolis, B.L., Kroes, W.H. & Quinn, R.P. (1974), "Job Stress: An Unlisted Occupational Hazard," *Journal of Occupational Medicine*, 16(10), 654-661.

National Safety News (1984), "Quick Return to Work Can Save Industry Millions," September, 51-52.

Patterson, D. (1986), "Determining Cost Benefits of Worksite Wellness," *Business and Health*, (October): 40-41.

Public Health Reports (1987), "Employers See Worksite Benefits in Health Promotion and Disease Prevention," Vol. 102: 457-458.

Pyle, R.L. (1979), "Corporate Fitness Programs—How Do They Shape Up?" *Personnel*, (Jan-Feb).

Schwartz, G.E. (1980), "Stress Management in Occupational Settings," *Public Health Reports*, (March-April) Vol. 95, No. 2: 99-108.

Shepard, D.S. and Pearlman, L.A. (1985), "Healthy Habits That Pay Off," *Business and Health,* 2,4 (March): 37-41.

Smith, K.J. (1987), "A Framework for Appraising," *Internal Auditor,* (December): 28-33.

Wagel, W.H. (1989), "Employee Wellness: TIAA-CREF's Rx for Good Living," *Personnel,* 66(1), 7-9.

Welling, K.M. (1990), "The Sickening Spiral," *Barron's,* Vol. LXX, No. 24, (June 11): 8-20.

ADOLESCENTS AS A PREVENTION AND INTERVENTION MARKET

Identifying and Reaching At-Risk Adolescents

Norm Bryan

Approximately twenty percent of adolescents in the United States are emotionally disturbed to some degree. Nationally, twelve percent of adolescents are estimated to fall into a dysfunctional category and are in need of mental health services (Davis, Kercheck & Schricker, 1986). An additional fifteen percent are vulnerable for developing a serious mental health problem (Davis et al., 1986). These are adolescents who are functioning at a minimum level and who are at a very high risk of becoming dysfunctional in times of stress.

Research on at-risk adolescents and mental health is increasingly focusing on adolescent suicide. Today, suicide by gunshot, drug overdose and a variety of other methods is the second leading cause of death among teenagers. It is occurring with greater frequency, particularly in the 15 to 19 year age group (Crumley, 1990). Acknowledging that the increased rate of suicide is partly a result of

Norm Bryan is affiliated with the Department of Management at Georgia State University.

127

more accurate reporting, Patros and Shamoo (1989) and Poland (1989) argue that suicidal behavior has reached critical proportions among youth and that intervention programs should be implemented. Thus, this paper first examines those factors associated with suicide including self-esteem, depression, and substance use. Second, given that intervention is critical for at-risk youths, methods of communicating with these individuals are discussed. Specifically, who is the most appropriate change agent and what is the most effective format to use to reach these individuals?

BACKGROUND

Adolescent suicide is a tragedy that has received much attention over the past several years, partially because of the increased number of suicides among adolescents. The suicide rate for white male adolescents aged 15 through 19 years increased 305 per cent from 1950 through 1980, while the rate for females increased almost 68 per cent during the same time period (Centers for Disease Control, 1986). The increase in youth suicide is due primarily to an increasing suicide rate among males. The suicide rate for males increased from 3.5 per 100,000 in 1950 to 13.8 per 100,000 in 1980, while for females the increase was from 1.8 per 100,000 in 1950 to 3.0 per 100,000 in 1980 (Centers for Disease Control, 1986).

Depression

Suicide has been related to depression, which has recently been recognized by the American Psychiatric Association as a psychopathological syndrome of children as well as adults. The rates of depression have increased for all those individuals born after 1940, with depression more often occurring during adolescence and young adulthood, rather than later in life (Klerman & Weissman, 1989). Depression may well be manifested in a student's expression of sadness, hopelessness and self-deprecation, withdrawal, changes in eating and sleeping patterns, and drug and alcohol use.

Substance abuse (both drug and alcohol) in adolescence has been linked with depression, conduct and personality disorders (see Crumley, 1990 for a comprehensive review). One or more of these combinations of disorders are often part of the description of the suicidal teenager. Crumley (1981) found that the effect of intoxication by alcohol or drugs seemed to deepen depression, which precipitated a suicide attempt. Moreover, substance abuse aggravated social or interpersonal problems which added to the depression in the long run.

Although gender differences in depression have not been heavily researched, self-acknowledged rates of depression are consistently lower for males than for females who are reported to have a greater lifetime risk of depression (Klerman & Weissman, 1989). Klerman (1988) noted that the rates for depression, suicide attempts/deaths, and drug abuse have all increased between 1960 and 1980. According to Klerman (1988), "There are important gender and ethnic differences in these rates: females are more prone to depression whereas males are more prone to suicide and drug abuse."

To summarize, studies suggest that adolescents who abuse drugs are more frequently troubled by suicidal thoughts, sadness, and emotional disturbances than are adolescents in general. Members of this population may also have had a previous suicide attempt or drug overdose episode. The rate of completed suicide appears to be higher in this population than in the general adolescent population (Crumley, 1990).

Crumley (1990) specifically examined the relationship between substance abuse and adolescent suicidal behavior. He reports that abuse of psychoactive substances appears to be associated with a greater frequency and number of suicide attempts, more suicidal thoughts and more serious intention, and a greater chance of more lethal attempts. Studies have also found a specific link between alcohol intoxication and suicide by gun shot among teenagers. Adolescents who use drugs, especially those who suffer from depression, appear to be at increased risk for suicidal behavior. Since research supports the association between drug use, depression and suicidal behavior, a brief examination of drug use among adolescents is warranted.

Drug Use

Alcohol and drug use is an issue that cannot be avoided. Teenagers will have both the opportunity and the inducement to use alcohol and/or other drugs. Alcohol is the most commonly abused drug among adolescents. Roughly 66% of seniors in the class of 1985 reported using alcohol in the past month with about one in 20 seniors using alcohol on a daily basis (National Institute on Drug Abuse, NIDA, 1986).

Alcohol use may begin at an early age. By 8th grade, approximately 30% had used alcohol, by 9th grade over 50% had used alcohol, by 10th grade, 75% had become users and by 12th grade over 92% had used the drug (NIAAA, 1983; NIDA, 1986). In general, experimentation with alcohol is beginning at an earlier age. Oetting and Beauvais (1990) in a comprehensive summary of the findings of national surveys on adolescent drug use report the following important patterns of adolescent drug use. First, there is some drug use among very young children. Although the rates are low, counselors and teachers should be aware that drug use does occur in the fourth to sixth grades. Also noted is that while marijuana is seen as the "gateway" drug, almost twice as many sixth graders had tried inhalants. Second, Oetting and Beauvais (1990) report considerable increases in use from the sixth to the ninth grades, indicating that this might be a vulnerable age for introduction to drug use. Substantial developmental changes occurring at this time as well as the transition from elementary school to junior high, middle school and high school could effect drug use.

A social stress model of substance abuse (Rhodes & Jason, 1990) posits that one of the contributing factors to drug use in adolescents is self-esteem. According to this model, adolescents initiate substance abuse as a means of coping with a variety of stressors and influences that may stem from within the family, the school, the peer group or the community.

A number of other studies have reported that in addition to the social influence of parents, family and peers, low self-esteem, low self-satisfaction, low self-confidence and high anxiety are correlated with substance abuse behavior (Orlandi, Dozier, & Martin, 1990). An understanding of the correlates, especially as they relate to the onset of substance abuse behavior would have a great influence on the development of interventions designed as primary prevention strategies (Botvin, 1986).

To summarize, the initiation of drug use occurs during adolescence and is the result of a combination of cognitive, attitudinal, social, personality, pharmacologic and developmental factors. For many individuals, the use of drugs is limited to a brief period of experimentation. For some individuals, however, experimentation with tobacco, alcohol or other drugs results in compulsive patterns of use which can lead to academic, social and emotional problems and interfere with normal psychosocial development (Botvin, Baker, Dusenbury, Tortu & Bovin, 1990).

Given that research has established a link between substance abuse, depression, self-esteem and suicide, it is important to examine how one can communicate with this subset of the adolescent population. Are some vehicles more effective than others in reaching these at-risk individuals? Are there predictable crisis and intervention points? Are some formats used in communicating with these individuals better than others? This study attempts to address these questions.

METHODOLOGY

The methodology used in this study consisted of the development of the research design, the data collection method, sampling, analysis and interpretation.

Research Design

This is a descriptive study of self-reported behavior. Written questionnaires were answered in a classroom setting. The questions were structured and the purpose of the questionnaire was not disguised. The questionnaires included items relating to drug use, self concept and sources of assistance and were administered to adolescents in grades five through twelve.

Data Collection Method

A short introductory comment was read to each classroom and the student interviewer read through the questionnaire with students making the appropriate responses. The questionnaires were gathered in a manila envelope; emphasis on security of information was thus maintained with students not being able to see the answers of others. Additionally, the field workers administering the questionnaire were upperclassmen of the school system to encourage students to answer honestly since their teachers would not be involved in handling the surveys.

Sampling

Approximately forty classes were randomly chosen using a two-stage cluster technique. From each grade one-half of the homeroom classes were chosen. Since the researchers had no reason to believe that the students in a particular class were more homogeneous in important personal characteristics than the overall population, this method should be as efficient as simple random sampling.

Analysis and Interpretation

The questionnaire asked the students to describe drug and alcohol consumption in terms of usage: daily, weekly, monthly, annually, have tried, and have not tried. Students also responded to the following three questions with a 5-item response format anchored with (1) almost always and (5) almost never: (1) Do you feel good about yourself?; (2) Do you feel depressed about life?; and (3) During the past year have you considered committing suicide? Finally, students were asked to indicate who during the past year they went to when they had problems (teacher, friend, coach, doctor, minister, parent, brother or sister, counselor, or kept it to myself) and the best method to use to communicate with them (classroom discussion, lecturer from outside the school, films, student led program, at home with parents, and reading material).

The self-report drug usage variables were summed across individuals to form three scales: Alcohol (consisting of beer, wine and liquor), Drugs (consisting of cocaine, crack, stimulants, marijuana, tranquilizers, PCP, opiates and hallucinogens) and Tobacco (Cigarettes and chewing tobacco/snuff). Ranges for the three scales are as follows: Alcohol (0-15), Drug (0-40) and Tobacco (0-10). Higher numbers on the scale indicate higher frequency of use.

These three scales (Alcohol, Drug and Tobacco) were used in a multivariate analysis of variance (MANOVA) to determine if differences in alcohol, drug and tobacco use were associated with different levels of depression, self-esteem, and suicidal thoughts. That is, do depressed individuals tend to use these substances more than individuals who are not depressed? Do adolescents who feel good about themselves use alcohol, drugs and tobacco in the same frequency as those adolescents who do not feel good about themselves? Do students with more suicidal thoughts use substances more than other students?

Chi-square analysis was used to detect whether or not significant differences existed among groups of individuals in terms of (1) the potential change agent, and (2) communication formats. That is, are certain change agents and communication formats more effective when communicating with at-risk individuals than the general adolescent population?

Limitations

Several possible factors may influence the results found in this study, particularly the factual nature of the answers. First, respondents may be unable to provide the information desired because of the difficulty in separating the original five levels of usage in the minds of the respondents. Second, the respondents may be unwilling to provide the information. For this reason, their peers were used to collect and seal the information, limiting "authority" figures from seeing the data. A third possible limiting factor is that the questioning process may stimulate incorrect or misleading answers; the nature of the topic may cause some amount of untruthfulness. However, Oetting and Beauvais (1990) contend that self-report among adolescents is likely to be reasonably trustworthy. Similarly, the required presence of the teacher in the classroom may influence answers, although the teachers did not have access to the questionnaires.

FINDINGS

Three scales (Alcohol, Drugs and Tobacco) were formed by summing variables across individuals. Cronbach alpha reliabilities for the three scales are .80, .86, and .54 respectively. Ranges, averages and standard deviations for the three scales are presented in Table 1. These scales represent drug use, alcohol use and tobacco use.

TABLE 1. Means, Standard Deviations and Ranges for the Alcohol, Drug, and Tobacco Scales

Scale	Range	Mean	Std. Deviation
Drugs	0-40	8.640	2.69
Alcohol	0-15	6.43	3.71
Tobacco	0-10	3.35	2.31

Multivariate Analysis of Variance Results

The MANOVA for self-esteem was not significant. That is, results performed on the entire sample indicate that there were no differences in alcohol, drug or tobacco use for individuals who felt good about themselves versus those individuals who did not.

Results of the MANOVA for depression indicate that there is a significant difference in drug use between depressed adolescents and those who are not depressed; depressed individuals report higher drug usage than individuals who are not depressed ($F = 16.07$; $p = .0001$). Alcohol and tobacco use for individuals who were depressed versus those who were not depressed did not differ significantly.

MANOVA results show that those individuals with higher thoughts of considering suicide in the past year had a significantly higher consumption of drugs ($F = 5.97$; $p = .015$), alcohol ($F = 14.03$, $p = .0001$) and tobacco ($F = 12.66$, $p = .0001$).

A MANOVA was also performed on the entire sample based upon three grade groupings: fifth through sixth grades, seventh through ninth grades, and tenth through twelfth grades to determine whether or not there were significant differences among these three groups in terms of alcohol and drug use. Results indicated that usage does vary by grade level. Further analysis though Scheefe's multiple comparison tests indicated that there is significantly more alcohol consumption in the seventh through ninth grades than in the fifth and sixth grades, and significantly more alcohol use in the tenth and twelfth grades than in the seventh through ninth grades. Multiple comparison tests on drug use revealed that significantly more drug use is taking place in the tenth to twelfth grades than in either of the other two groups.

Chi-Square Analysis of Sources of Help and Communication Format

Table 2 presents percentages for the entire sample (n = 931) in terms of who individuals went to during the past year when they had problems. Friends were the primary source of support and help for the entire sample (60.8%), with parents following second (51.7%). Interestingly, half of the sample (50.5%) used themselves for guidance on problems. However, teachers, counselors, and ministers/priests had low utilization rates, 12.8%, 8.8%, and 6.9% respectively.

TABLE 2. Reference Groups and Communication Channels Preferences for the Entire Sample

<u>Usage of Individuals for Guidance on Problems</u>

Friend	60.8%
Parent	51.7%
Self	50.5%
Sibling	28.3%
Teacher	12.8%
Counselor	8.8%
Coach	6.9%
Minister/Priest	6.9%
Doctor	5.1%

Also presented in Table 2 are the most preferred methods of addressing crucial issues. Students felt that the school situation is the most effective method for addressing social issues with over 51% proposing classroom discussion with teachers and 45% listing films. Reading material was seen as the least effective method of addressing crucial issues (19%). To learn more about how to communicate with potentially at-risk adolescents, chi-square analysis was used to determine whether significant differences existed between students based upon self-esteem, depression, and suicidal thoughts. That is, do depressed youths or adolescents with thoughts of suicide differ from the overall sample in terms of who they go to for help, or in their preferred communication format?

Results of the chi-square analysis of who individuals go to for help indicate that adolescents who felt good about themselves (high self-esteem) differ significantly in two ways from those who do not feel good about themselves (low self-esteem). First, high self-esteem individuals tend to turn to parents more than low self-esteem students ($p = .01$). Second, those youths with low self-esteem turn more to themselves in time of trouble than do youths with high self-esteem ($p = .001$). There were no significant differences for these groups in terms of communication formats; both high self-esteem and low self-esteem individuals reported the same preferences for addressing critical issues.

Three significant differences emerged when the sample was analyzed based upon individuals who reported being depressed versus those who experienced little to no depression. First, depressed adolescents turn to their parents less often in times of trouble than do youths who reported experiencing less depression ($p = .005$). Second, depressed individuals are more likely to turn to themselves in time of need than do those reporting little or no depression ($p = .004$). Third, depressed adolescents report a higher incidence of talking to their doctor than do other individuals ($p = .008$). There were no significant differences for these groups in terms of communication formats.

Finally, three differences were present between individuals who had considered thoughts of suicide fairly often versus those who had never or only rarely had suicidal thoughts. First, those individuals reporting suicidal thoughts reported talking to pastors more often than did the other group (p = .01). Second, those with suicidal thoughts are much less likely to turn to their parents than are those youths with rare thoughts of suicide (p = .001). Third, individuals with more suicidal thoughts reported talking to their school counselors more than did students with few thoughts of suicide (p = .0001). When the preferred formats for communicating with students were examined, the only way in which this group differed significantly from other students, was that they did not prefer the format of being home with their parents as a way to receive information (p = .001). While not significant (p = .16), students with suicidal thoughts were less likely to prefer classroom discussions with the teacher as a way of addressing critical issues.

While few differences were present when the preferred communication format was examined by self-esteem, depression, and suicide, significant differences did emerge when the formats were examined by grade and gender. In general, females at all grade levels preferred discussing topics with their teacher in a classroom setting more than male students (p = .0004).

Discussion or counseling with the teacher appears to be a more effective format when utilized in the early grades (fifth and sixth) than in later grades (p = .0001). While counseling with friends is not important in the early grades (fifth and sixth), it becomes increasingly important as the student becomes older and progresses through the school system (p = .0001). Counseling with parents is preferred by younger students (fifth and sixth grades), and becomes increasingly less preferred as the student is in higher grades, particularly the junior and senior years of high school (p = .0001).

When the communication format was analyzed by grade, it seems that outside lecturers are preferred in the tenth, eleventh and twelfth grades (p = .0002), while films are more popular with younger grades such as the eighth and ninth grades (p = .026). Students also start preferring student led programs around the eighth and ninth grades (p = .029). Reading material is also preferred more in the lower grades (fifth through the eight) than in the higher grades (p = .001).

RECOMMENDATIONS

Several implications stem from the results presented. First, the multivariate analysis of variance demonstrated that drug use is associated with depression. Although causality was not determined, it is shown that higher drug use is associated with higher levels of depression. Second, drug, alcohol, and tobacco consumption are associated with thoughts of suicide. Students who have more thoughts of suicide have greater consumption of these substances.

The chi-square analysis demonstrated that individuals who are depressed, have low self-esteem and have though about suicide in the past year are less likely to turn to their parents for support and guidance than are adolescents in general. Thus, trying to reach these individuals through parents and through in-home activities may not be effective.

REFERENCES

Botvin, G. J. (1986). Substance abuse prevention research; Recent developments and future directions. *Journal of School Health, 56,* 369-374.

Botvin, G. J., Baker, E., Dusenbury, L., Tortu, S., & Bovin, E. (1990). Preventing adolescent drug abuse through a multimodal cognitive-behavioral approach: Results of a 3-year study. *Journal of Consulting and Clinical Psychology, 58,* 437-446.

Crumley, F. E. (1981). Adolescent suicide attempts and borderline personality disorder. *Southern Medical Journal, 74,* 546-549.

Crumley, F. E. (1990). Substance abuse and adolescent suicidal behavior. *Journal of the American Medical Association, 263,* 3051-3056.

Davis, M. F., Kercheck, B. A., & Schricker, B. J. (1986). *Adolescent health in Colorado: Status, Implications and Strategies for Action.* Denver: Advisory Council on Adolescent Health, Colorado Department of Health.

Klerman, G. J. (1988). The current age of youthful melancholie: evidence for increase in depression among adolescents and young adults. *British Journal of Psychiatry, 152,* 4-14.

Klerman, G. J., & Weissman, M. M. (1989). Increasing rates of depression. *Journal of the American Medical Association, 261,* 2229-2235.

National Institute on Alcohol Abuse and Alcoholism. (1983). *Alcohol and Health.* Washington, D.C.: Department of Health and Human Services.

National Institute on Drug Abuse. (1986). *Drugs and American high school students.* Washington, D.C.: Department of Health and Human Services.

Oetting, E. R., & Beauvais, F. (1990). Adolescent drug use: Findings of national and local surveys. *Journal of Consulting and Clinical Psychology, 58,* 385-394.

Orlandi, M. A., Dozier, C. E., & Martin, M. A. (1990). Computer-Assisted Strategies for Substance Abuse Prevention: Opportunities and Barriers. *Journal of Counseling and Clinical Psychology, 58,* 425-431.

Patros, P.G., & Shamoo, T. K. (1989). *Depression and suicide in children and adolescents: Prevention, intervention, and postvention.* Boston: Allyn and Bacon.

Poland, S. (1989). *Suicide Intervention in the Schools.* New York: Guilford.

Rhodes, J. E., & Jason, L. A. (1990). A Social stress model of substance abuse. *Journal of Consulting and Clinical Psychology, 58,* 395-401.

Youth Suicide in the United States, 1970-1980. (1986). Atlanta, GA: Centers for Disease Control.

SOME MARKETING TOOLS: BUILDING A MARKETING ENVIRONMENT, PROMOTION AND EVALUATION

Reports from the Field: Building a Marketing Environment in Community Mental Health Settings

Susannah Grimm Poe

SUMMARY. Many non-profit mental health centers have been slow to embrace a market-driven approach to service delivery. This article explains how those organizations can begin to develop a market orientation through an easy to follow, step by step process that begins with a commitment to audience needs and wants, builds on do-it-yourself market research, and culminates in a viable marketing plan.

Marketing used to be one of the most powerful words you could say in mental health settings. Just mentioning the "M" word emptied entire rooms of staffers.

Susannah Grimm Poe, AMHC, MSJ, LSW, is Director of Marketing and Training at the Summit Center for Human Development, 6 Hospital Plaza, Clarksburg, WV 26301.

141

Those who refused the idea of marketing years ago, however, have been replaced by battle-weary veterans of retrenchments, shifting priorities, and overload, who have learned the hard way that the dreaded "M" word had a very useful role in their survival. This attitude change mirrors the financial history of the community mental health movement (Okin 1984). Though fully funded with federal dollars in its flush early years, now community mental health faces ever decreasing government support. The once favored child must now scramble to survive, and that translates, in part, to marketing.

And those reluctant mental health professionals are not alone. Since Kotler, Levy, Zaltman, and Shapiro first described the phenomenon of social marketing in the late 60's and early 70's, health care professionals have embraced the promise, if not the experience, of marketing their not-for-profit services (Kotler and Andreasen 1990).

One of the most obvious illustrations of this acceptance is the fact that mental health centers, following the lead of hospitals, have begun to embrace marketing as a viable means by which their organization could compete in an increasingly sophisticated environment — an environment where the customer or customers drives the service.

Marketing is still a powerful word in mental health centers, but this time it's a promise instead of a threat.

Even with marketing in a new light, most clinical and support staff of mental health centers don't know what marketing is, how to market, and especially don't know how powerful a role they play in the success of any organizational marketing effort.

Marketing is an integrated effort to enhance the positive image, visibility, and approachability of your organization to those you serve and to encourage that public to render any support necessary for survival. Simplified, marketing is an EXCHANGE — we provide access to mental health services that you need and want, and you help us continue doing so.

Your first job as a marketer, then, is to determine how ready your organization is to become market-driven. Does your staff have a grasp of the exchange involved in marketing, or does it still equate marketing with selling and advertising: a "here it is, come and get it" mentality?

Does your staff realize that everyone in the organization is a marketer, and that how well they meet the needs of their clients is in direct relation to how long they'll stay in business?

There are four stages in the marketing growth of any organization. The first three: product orientation, production orientation, and selling orientation, are characterized by management placing the needs and desires of the organization in the center of the strategic planning process (Schulman 1987). "It is only when management realizes that it is the customer who truly determines the long-run success of any strategy that the non-profit firm can join the ranks of the sophisticated customer-centered marketing strategists typically found in the private sector" (Kotler and Andreasen 1990).

Is your staff and management truly interested in what clients — both internal and external — want and desire? Are they willing to undertake and then respond to audience feedback?

It is serious and respectful attention from staff members at every level of the organization to consumer needs and wants, and a commitment to deliver services tailored to those needs and wants, that signals your organization is ready to begin serious marketing.

Make sure it is the commitment to the customer, not the desire to embrace a popular buzzword, that's behind the demand for marketing.

But once the organization is moving toward that customer orientation, it's our task as mental health marketers to infuse enough marketing know-how into the organizational culture to help those staffers understand and "own" the marketing of their services. They need to know the steps in a viable market plan: the mission statement, segmentation of audiences, gathering audience feedback, and developing a marketing plan that incorporates that mission and audience feedback.

But how do you take a staff of converted believers and provide them with the skill and knowledge that will encourage them to adopt the above marketing steps? Further, how do you do accomplish that marketing awareness and ownership with a minimal budget, little staff training time and/or hands-on inclination for marketing education?

How? Begin by asking the staff you're serving what they need and want to know about marketing, and then deliver that help. It might be the loan of a textbook (such as Kotler and Andreasen's new edition of *Strategic Marketing for Nonprofit Organizations*), or the sharing of some good marketing articles, or even a short course on marketing — but by letting your staff, the internal audience, determine what they need, you are demonstrating true marketing strategy from step one.

However you arrive at it, your goal is to increase the practical marketing knowledge of all members of the organization in a way they can understand and make it work for them.

Once a basic understanding of marketing is embraced by all staff, the next step is to begin the work of defining your organization's mission through feedback from your internal audience.

THE MISSION STATEMENT

Ask your staff about the reason they work in mental health, how they feel about their work, the clients, and the organization. Find out their concerns and their beliefs, and how they feel the organization contributes to those concerns and beliefs.

That information becomes the basis of your mission statement. The statement must be concise, viable, motivating, and personalized, and should suggest the values and goals of the internal audience.

> A mission statement has to be operational, otherwise it's just good intentions. A mission statement has to focus on what the institution really tries to do and then do it so that everybody in the organization can say, 'This is my contribution to the goal.' (Drucker 1990)

The mission statement, if it accurately records the pulse of the organization, will be the cornerstone of all the marketing and planning to come. It is your organizational reason-to-be. Post it everywhere — it reflects the conscience and purpose of your organization.

SEGMENTING YOUR AUDIENCES

Once we have developed an understanding of who we are, the next step is to understand who we serve.

Understanding who we serve, how effectively we serve them,

and how we can maximize continued service delivery are critical survival questions in today's non-profit environment. Having the real answers to those questions — answers that make sense to you, your Board, and your public, is the cornerstone of marketing mental health — and the key to staying in business.

Who we serve, in marketing terms, is known as our "audience." Mental health service providers, like all human service organizations, have three major audiences: external, channel members, and internal.

Each of those audiences has a critical and differing role in the EXCHANGE that means our survival. Each audience requires a different service (or product) from us, and the satisfaction of each audience depends on how well we understand and deliver what they need.

Our ongoing understanding of the needs of our varied audiences — and segments of those audiences (through audience surveying), our ability to satisfy those needs (service delivery), and finally our expertise at delivering and communicating that satisfactory relationship (public relations) are components of successful marketing plans (Stone, Warren, and Stevens 1990).

The most easily identified mental health center audience, of course, is our primary client or clients . . . the individual or family with a behavioral health concern that causes them to seek relief through our professional services. Surrounding that primary client is his or her extended family, employers, and neighbors — a critical audience to our organization for two reasons. First, their understanding and endorsement of that therapy or treatment has an impact on its success, and secondly because word-of-mouth recommendation is a major persuader to those considering mental health services (Poe 1990; Gubman and Tessler 1987; Lefley 1989; Wahl and Harman 1989). That client and his or her support system is part of our EXTERNAL AUDIENCE.

Also included in the external category are our potential clients: those folks out there that we know statistically (and anecdotally if you've ever worked crisis intervention on Friday closing time) are at risk.

Add to that external category all those nameless and faceless folks who never walk through our doors but whose good will and understanding of our services is critical to positive word-of-mouth support and community acceptance.

The second major audience category is that of CHANNEL MEMBER. A channel member is someone who refers, oversees, manages, observes, or funds your organization but is not on your organization's payroll. Channel members may be officers of the court who refer clients for assessment, or a board member, or a television reporter who knows to call for a comment when someone plunges from a local bridge. This audience has a greater knowledge or interest in your service delivery system because they "channel" desired resources (clients, operating funds, good word-of-mouth, publicity) toward your organization.

The third audience of mental health services is INTERNAL—every member of your organization. Last thought of, often, but certainly not least, this audience segment is most critical to the success of our service delivery. How they feel about their work and the work of their peers at the front desk and down the hall is often overlooked in audience surveying, but primary to the success of all marketing efforts.

GAINING AUDIENCE FEEDBACK

Remember that in a true market-driven organization, the critical questions are: What do our audience members want? How are we doing at providing that service? What can we do to improve their satisfaction? (Kirchner 1981).

Once you've begun segmenting your audiences and understanding each segment's unique importance to your survival, you can ask each for feedback that will shape the future of your organization.

Begin by considering these four points:

1. Know what questions you want answered before you begin. Then tailor your questions to each audience in a way that will have the best chance of being answered.

As you begin market surveying, you will most likely want to know what your audiences know about your organization, how well they think your organization is performing its work, and what could be improved. You might also want to know how your clients and the public regard your organization, staff, location, pricing, and facilities. Be sure to ask enough demographic information (age, gender, race, income, etc.) to help profile the specific audience and then maybe better understand their responses based on that profile.

Of course, you will develop each survey to fit the specific audience, keeping in mind their overall knowledge of your organization, their education level, and their ability to understand and provide you with needed feedback.

Make sure you include similar questions, though, for each audience. You may want to ask your staff "What's the mission of _____?" while you ask a client "What do you think is the purpose of our organization?" Though not alike word for word, the responses to that question about mission can be compared for interesting results.

Another answer that can easily be compared is your staff's response to "Where do you think our clients first hear about our services?" while you ask the client "Where did you first hear of our services?" Similar questions asked to different audiences and then compared will provide you with information about how well your internal and external audience understand one another.

2. You have to know what you're going to do with the information you receive and, especially, make a commitment to use it in a positive way. The most anti-marketing move you can make is to ask for feedback you're not going to use, or decide not to use the feedback you receive because you don't agree with it.

3. You need to acknowledge the exchange involved in this feedback exercise. If you ask your audiences to help you, what can you give them in return for their help? Perhaps in exchange for their time and answers you can show them survey results, or provide lunch, or make a commitment to positive change based on their answers. But you owe them something for their ideas.

4. How can you find out what you want to know from each particular audience, and do so in a dignified, valid, and confidential (if applicable) manner. In other words, what feedback tool can you use?

Two inexpensive, reliable, relatively simple, and satisfying methods of finding out what your audience thinks, wants, and needs are through written surveys and focus groups.

WRITTEN SURVEYS

Audience surveying through a written questionnaire, either with an entire population (like staff) or a sampling (every client who comes for services during one week), can provide interesting and measurable feedback.

When designing your questionnaire, keep in mind these three rules: make sure you have a good reason for asking each question, keep it short and simple, and pretest it with a small sample of the audience before using it (Steiber 1988).

Attempt to limit systemic bias, which will prevent a representative response. That means, among other things, that you must consider the non-readers, or those who can't hear or write, by providing assistance in completing the survey. Make sure the entire sample has an equal opportunity to participate, and that all who chose to participate have adequate time to respond.

The sample size is also important. Generally, the larger the sample the more accurate the information, because you have more direct response from audience members. But a small representative sample can also provide valid results. The decision of sample size must be based on what you know, and want to know, of the audience.

Say you want to measure the satisfaction of your present outpatient client population. Since outpatient clients are generally seen once a week, or every other week, and equal numbers are seen every day of the week and across all time slots, you could select one week each month to ask every outpatient client who comes in for an appointment to fill out the survey. You then have a sample size of approximately one-fourth to one-half of your audience. If you ran the survey for a continuous two week period, or even for a month, you would run the risk of duplicating client response.

On the other hand, when surveying staff (of a manageable size) you could use the entire audience because they are an audience of fixed number who stay in one place most of the time.

Your questions should be user friendly, both for the respondents and for the software program you will be using to compile results. Remember when you pretest to enter responses into the computer — and pull out the info you'll be seeking — to make sure your questionnaire will be workable. In more "hands-on" centers, design the survey for the ease of the respondent and the analyst who will compile the results by hand.

Should your answer format be open ended or scaled? Again, this depends on who you're asking and what information you're seeking. Open-ended questions usually provide interesting anecdotal responses, but are often difficult to measure against other responses to the same question. Yes or no answers are easy to quantify, but don't provide for the "sometimes yes, sometimes no" answers your respondent might prefer. "Questions with a Likert response format are easier for the respondent and the analyst. Usually coded along the lines of 'very satisfied,' 'somewhat satisfied,' 'neutral,' 'somewhat dissatisfied,' 'very dissatisfied,' they capture two desirable attributes" of a conceptual midpoint (neutral) and the same number of choices on either side of neutral (Steiber 1989).

FOCUS GROUPS

Focus groups are an excellent way to get an in-depth look at how a certain audience segment perceives your services. This method of audience research works particularly well with internal audiences and channel members.

A focus group is a gathering of 7-10 people who represent the audience segment you're studying. They are interviewed by an impartial facilitator during a comfortable period of time usually ranging from an hour to two hours. Refreshments are usually available before and sometimes during the session to encourage an informal, relaxed environment.

The facilitator begins by explaining the reason for the focus group (like the organization wants to know how members of the community perceive mental health care). He or she describes the **focus group** as an opportunity for the decision-makers of the sponsoring organization to learn more about the opinions of that group and those they represent.

If the session is to be audiotaped for later transcription, the facilitator explains that process to the assembled group. Sometimes audiences are videotaped or viewed through a two-way mirror, and if that's the case the participants must be informed of this—and the reasons for it (often to gain insight from body language)—before they begin.

Participants are then given friendly ground rules. They are encouraged to speak one at a time, and distinctly enough for the recording. They are told there are no right or wrong answers—all responses are valuable to the organization. And they are introduced to the topic by the facilitator, who explains his or her role is to ask questions and prompt discussion.

Often the facilitator concludes this general introduction with a personal introduction, and invites everyone else to do the same. In situations when the confidentiality of the participant's opinion might be a concern (perhaps when internal staff discuss organizational improvements), allow everyone to adopt false names. In these special cases, you can ask the facilitator to provide a transcription of proceedings and to present an overview of the discussion, sans identities. Of course, you would not videotape this audience.

The facilitator has a preplanned set of questions which, like written surveys, are carefully designed to answer questions that will help you better understand your audiences and their needs. You may also want to test the value of your service, or product, by asking the group's opinion.

Be careful in your choice of facilitator. You need to have someone uninvolved in the topic of the focus group, so that he or she won't consciously or unconsciously bias the discussion. "The choice of this person is critical: A poor moderator can waste time, allow the group to be influenced by dominant participants, and permit the session to create more problems than it sets out to solve" (Smith 1982).

Holding multiple focus groups with different audiences but using the same questionnaire will increase the validity of your findings. Points raised by all groups are, of course, most reliable. Be sure to use the same facilitator, and accommodations for each group, to insure the closest reliability of results.

USING THE RESULTS
OF YOUR AUDIENCE FEEDBACK

Now is the time for truth or consequences.

You have the data "truth" that you need to begin customer-driven marketing. Audience opinion of your organization and its products has been gleaned from inside and out. You should have a better idea of who your customers are and what they want from your organization.

Make sure every decision-maker in your organization (and isn't that everyone?) has access to the marketing survey results. Prepare a compilation of results for your management team, discuss the results at your staff meetings, publish results in your newsletter, present your findings to your Board. Knowledge is truly power when it comes to marketing.

Then each segment of your organization, from management team to support services, must take the overall mission statement and the compiled audience feedback and build unit by unit an outline for services that incorporates what the organization stands for and what the audience wants and needs.

This outline for service delivery must now consider McCarthy's four P's of marketing: product, price, placement, and promotion (McCarthy and Perreault, 1984).

The "product" in mental health organizations is, generally, a *service* like outpatient therapy. The product is what the customers have told you they want or need, and what they are willing to exchange their resources (of money or good word-of-mouth, for example) to receive. The product will be different for each part of your organization. A children's developmental disabilities program will have a different service to offer clients than the professionals who service the chronically mentally ill clients. That is why it is important for each member of your organization to have a grasp of marketing skills, so that they can create the best exchange for their audience segment and, in turn, support the whole.

"Pricing" the service depends on three factors: what the customer is willing to pay, what the organization needs to survive, and how competitive that price is within the community. It is simply the rate of exchange. The customer is willing to pay so much of their desired resource for your product or service, and you're willing and able to accept that amount. Ask too much than the client is willing to pay and you won't serve that client. Charge less than it takes you to provide the service and you won't stay in business.

"Placement," simplified, is where you are located, geographically and competitively. You must be in a location that can easily and comfortably accommodate your customers, and you must be visible and desirable in a market often packed with organizations offering what looks like the same service. Part of your marketing plan must be to seek the best placement so that customers may learn about your organization and avail themselves of your services.

One way you distinguish yourself is through your "promotion" activities, a.k.a. public relations and advertising. Here again your audience feedback provides an advantage: design products your target audiences want and need and then tell them about it, using the same terms and phrases they gave you when they described the desired service.

Using the terminology of the customer in developing an exchange they need or want is particularly important to the mental health marketer. Most mental health organizations sell intangible products, like therapy or day programming, that can't be seen or felt or easily explained to the potential consumer. Using words used by the clients to build your product, and then to explain it to them, adds some recognizable tangibility to your product. Other ideas to add dimension to intangible products are brochures, videos, logos, slogans, and testimonials.

Once you have developed the product the target customer needs or wants, tell them about it. Tell them about it over the television, through the newspaper, on the radio, at health fairs, at club meetings, in church, through workshops, anyway that you know how to best reach the audience you're aiming for. Remember that each audience has a preferred method of communications: your market research should help you define (remember the question asking "how did you first hear about us?") the way they can be reached. A retired audience, for example, may respond to an interview on the local noon news, while a working woman may hear you best via radio in the usual before and after work commuting hours.

A good marketing plan is a work in progress: flexible enough to meet the changing needs of each audience. It is written specifically enough to outline objectives and responsibilities, and to clarify budget and time frames. It takes into consideration the management style of the organization and allows each person to work in a way that is meaningful to him and the organization. Successful marketing plans are comprehensive, and include consideration of every segment of your internal and external audience.

But most of all, a good marketing plan is built on the needs and the desires of your audiences, both internal and external.

REFERENCES

Drucker, Peter F. (1990). *Managing the Nonprofit Organization,* New York: HarperCollins Publishers.

Gubman, Gayle D. and Richard C. Tessler (1987). "The Impact of Mental Illness on Families," *Journal of Family Issues,* 8 (2, June) 226-245.

Kirchner, John H. (1981). "Patient Feedback on Satisfaction with Direct Services Received at a Community Mental Health Center," *Psychotherapy: Theory, Research and Practice,* 18 (3, Fall), 359-364.

Kotler, Philip and Alan Andreasen (1990). *Strategic Marketing for Nonprofit Organizations,* New Jersey: Prentice-Hall.

Lefley, Harriet P. (1989). "Family Burden and Stigma in Major Mental Illness," *American Psychologist,* 44 (3), 556-559.

McCarthy, Jerome E. and William D. Perreault (1984). *Basic Marketing: A Managerial Approach,* Homewood, Ill.: Richard D. Irwin.

Okin, Robert L. (1984). "How Community Mental Health Centers are Coping," *Hospital and Community Psychiatry,* 35 (11, November) 1118-1128.

Poe, Susannah Grimm (1990). Unpublished results of client surveys, focus groups. Clarksburg, WV: Summit Center for Human Development.

Schulman, Jerome L. (1987). "The Transition from Clinician to Administrator to Marketer," *The Journal of Health Care Marketing,* 7 (4, December), 45-51.

Smith, Robert M. "Knowledge is Power: Research Can Help Your Marketing Program Succeed," *Case Currents,* (May/June 1982): 8-14.

Steiber, Steven R. "Preventing Pitfalls in Patient Surveys," *Health Care Strategic Management,* (May 1989): 13-16.

Stone, Terry R., William E. Warren and Robert E. Stevens (1990). "Segmenting the Mental Health Care Market," *Journal of Health Care Marketing,* 10 (1), 65-69.

Wahl, Otto F. and Charles R. Harman (1989). "Family Views of Stigma," *Schizophrenia Bulletin,* 15 (1), 131-138.

Building a Marketing Environment: A Case Study

Susannah Grimm Poe

Reading the mind of our community was the challenge Summit Center for Human Development faced more than two years ago when our management team was considering the merger of our out-patient services with the inpatient psychiatric unit of our local hospital.

To the management team (then comprised of Summit's executive director, associate director, fiscal director, medical director, and personnel director) the opportunities of such a merger seemed promising: increased community visibility, an opportunity to provide more comprehensive services to clients, and a strengthening of our position through an alliance with the major health care provider in our multi-count catchment area.

The drawbacks were also obvious: start up costs were previously unbudgeted, management of the combined unit could be threatening to our autonomy, and our own staff's concerns about the implications of such a merger could unravel the successful union.

Marketing, long a viable though underutilized part of Summit's infrastructure, was called upon to launch an extensive audience research project to add the consumer viewpoint to the decision-making process . . . to better understand our niche in the community and how it would be affected by such a merger, and, as importantly, to hear from our own staff about our present strengths and weaknesses and to learn their thoughts and concerns about the proposed merger.

Summit Center, a comprehensive community mental health cen-

Susannah Grimm Poe, AMHC, MSJ, LSW, is Director of Marketing and Training at the Summit Center for Human Development, 6 Hospital Plaza, Clarksburg, WV 26301.

ter serving citizens in five counties of north central West Virginia, had through the systematic education efforts of the executive director, approached the fourth stage of developing a marketing mindset and was being pulled, albeit kicking and screaming, into a customer centered orientation.

The commitment of the management team was real: marketing was given a permanent seat on the management team and the members agreed that the finding of the market research would help drive the decision-making process.

We began with what we considered our most immediately important and accessible audiences: the clients we were now serving and our own staff.

Written audience surveys and focus groups were our chosen methods of audience research. Both of these tools were quick and easy for us to use, and required little financial outlay.

Our first step of this planned effort was to survey our clients to find the reason for their visits to our center, what they wanted from their visit, how they first heard of Summit Center, how they first contacted Summit, if they were satisfied with the services they had received, what had been satisfying, what suggestions they had for improving our services, and demographic information including age, gender, payment category (including self pay and third party payers).

Every client who came through our doors during one week in February was given a survey to complete. This one sheet of questions began with an explanation of the survey and how the results would be used. The receptionist had the surveys attached to clipboards with a pen attached, and offered help in filling out the form if the client desired. Ninety clients completed the written survey, a response rate we calculated to be about 90 percent.

Those surveys were collected and compiled, and a written report was given to the management team, the staff, and the board of directors. Copies of the results were made available for staff.

Next, we circulated a two-paged questionnaire to all staff. This questionnaire was divided into two sections. The first dealt with **service delivery**: why staff thought clients came to Summit, what those clients desired as a result of their visit, did the staff think clients were satisfied with services, what specific comments could they recall from clients, and where did they think most clients first heard of Summit?

Section two dealt with the proposed merger. We asked staff to describe in their own words the purpose of the merger, when they thought it would occur, what they perceived their role to be in the merger (and if they were satisfied with that role), what additional information they needed to understand such a merger, and how satisfied they were generally with Summit's operations: internally, with clients, and with the general public.

These questions were chosen for several reasons. We wanted to know how well the management team was communicating the merger proposition to the general staff, what else we could provide to help them to understand and own the decision, and we wanted a bigger picture — what did they think of life as it was at Summit Center, in terms of client delivery systems and management success?

Implicit in this surveying was a clear and important message: we're in this together and we want to know what you think.

Required with this message was a promise: we'll let you know what we learn from this survey and incorporate it in the decision-making process. That promise, we considered, was critical to the success of our survey.

We launched the written survey on our monthly staff meeting day, when the largest contingent of staff is usually in one place. We put surveys in every staff member's mailbox, and made sure we had a few extras available. The survey was announced during the staff meeting, and staff were encouraged to complete the lengthy form that morning and place it in a designated mailbox. It was confidential in design, not requiring any identifying information.

The response rate was more than 75% of those staff attending the meeting that day, and about 25% of all staff.

Again, we compiled the findings and disseminated the information to the management team, the program managers, board of directors, and any staff who wanted to see the compilation.

Once we had surveyed a sampling of our clients and staff, we decided to ask members of our channel group and of the general public for feedback on Summit's products, placement, pricing, and promotion. We chose to utilize focus groups as the mechanism by which to listen to these groups.

The two channel member groups represented were managers from the hospital with whom we might merge and our own Board of Directors. The other four groups representing the general public included members of the county Extension Homemakers clubs, employees of a local utility company, members of the area Business and Professional Women's club, and a sampling of those receiving Aid to Families with Dependent Children (AFDC).

The outline for questioning each of these focus group audiences would be the same. We made a conscious decision not to ask any audience about the proposed merger, hoping to learn from the hospital and board representatives what they already, unprompted, knew about the proposal.

Focus group participants would be asked, hypothetically, for what reasons they would decide to seek mental health treatment, where would they go for treatment and what factors would influence that decision, what kind of services did they think we offered, what could Summit do to improve services to the community, what was a fair price for those services, and what did they think of our name and location.

Each group was invited to come to Summit at a certain time and was asked to wait in the lobby until we came for them. This was a short wait, but gave the participants time to experience the first stages of any client experience. Then we began the interview by asking how it felt to come to a mental health center. We found that question provided us with surprisingly good insight into our initial delivery system, and ALWAYS let to the issue of stigma — an issue we had not planned to raise.

Five of the six planned Focus Groups went off without a hitch. The sixth, the one comprised of AFDC recipients, was arranged through the local department of human services which, after agreeing to pull together such a group for us, decided that it couldn't be done due to confidentiality and transportation issues.

These external focus groups were led by a new member of Summit's marketing staff who had much previous experience as a group facilitator. We provided a healthy lunch to all participants, and gave each member of the group a flower from the centerpiece at the conclusion of the interview. We also wrote each a thank you note from the marketing director and from the executive director.

Because of the wealth of information we learned from our external focus groups, we decided to follow up our internal staff survey with three focus groups from our staff: one of middle managers and the other two comprised of randomly-selected staff representing all Summit programs.

A marketing expert with focus group experience was hired to help us conduct these internal discussion groups. We provided the same amenities as with our external groups: lunch, flowers, and thank you's.

Participants were asked questions similar to those contained in their staff survey, and responses from those surveys were shared with focus group members to provide a starting point for the discussion.

Although these discussions (like all our focus groups) were audiotaped for transcription, staff were assured that their anonymity would be guarded and were offered the opportunity to use a pseudonym during the discussion. Our external consultant handled the tapes and the transcription, providing us with typed copies of the proceeding sans names and identifying information. He also highlighted responses he considered as major themes and provided the management team with a written and oral report of the focus group findings. The results of these internal focus groups were also made available to staff.

What we learned was at once heartening, powerful, and challenging. We learned that there was an immense amount more to be learned. As in all good marketing, we raised more questions when we answered the first.

Specifically, we gained insight into how well our staff understood our present clients: their answers matched point to point the answers of clients on questions inquiring what clients wanted from Summit, their satisfaction level (very satisfied), what was satisfying (their interaction with our staff), and so on. Communications, internally and to the public, needed improvement, they urged. Tell us what we, as a center, do and keep us involved in the process. And, from a few, we received thanks from our staff for being asked.

We learned how our clients termed what they knew about us:

nice, caring people; professional and businesslike; located in a comfortable, clean setting. It was scary to come for help, we learned, but warm and satisfying when they began using our services. We found our clients wanted quick help, both in setting an appointment, in the waiting area, and once treatment began. They wanted more information about the treatment process, especially at the beginning.

Our channel members, we learned, sometimes had the greater problem with stigma than the remainder of our audiences. We found they sometimes lacked a clear picture of the comprehensiveness of our services. Many of them assigned services to our organization that was never, and could never, belong to us.

The general public groups told us that they would have to be at the end of their rope to go anywhere for treatment — unless their children or elderly parents needed help. The word of their minister or doctor, friends or family would help them decide if and then where they would seek treatment. They urged us to go into the community — to churches and club meetings and into the newspaper — with our message. Several members even disclosed, to our surprise, that they had been satisfied consumers of our services and would be willing to offer public testimonials on our behalf. They told us they were worried about school-aged children and self esteem and drugs; and that work stress was a problem for many of them. Many expected a different setting for mental health services than the bucolic location of Summit: there were comments on the peacefulness of our environment.

As we began to read the mind of our community, we learned much about ourselves and our mission. Most of what we learned was affirming, and seconded our often-voiced internal belief in the value of our mission. What was not positive was instructive, and has provided us with a roadmap for future travels.

We are committed to continuing the dialogue, and to act on the usefulness of this information with conscious planning.

Internally, the conversation continues. As a result of audience feedback, we have developed a staff newsletter that allows each department an opportunity to highlight its activities and gives management a chance to explain, clarify, and gain input into center policy.

As requested in focus groups, staff meetings have expanded to include reports from each department, and to affirm those who have supported the Center in a unique and valuable way during the past month.

We are in the process of another staff survey, similar to the first but adding questions on what we have accomplished in the past year and what remains to be accomplished. Our mission, as our feedback, is ever in process.

This staff survey will be followed by three more focus groups, two comprised of veterans of last year's efforts, and one of never-before participants. We will ask similar questions, and compare the responses from the first group to the second.

Our clients have been surveyed three times a year since the first survey in February, 1989. We have maintained much the same format, except to add satisfaction questions about our location, staff, and overall impression of our Center. We have also included a scale asking what clients wanted from their Center visit, from "quality of therapist" to "convenient location." (Quality of therapist always comes in first but raises the next generation of questions — how does that client DEFINE quality?)

Results of these client surveys are always given to the management team, our staff, and our Board, and are highlighted in our newsletter. Often, statistics from these surveys are quoted during our semi-weekly noon television interviews on a local channel.

One of the most positive and visible results these surveys have had is in affirming our staff. Each client survey has provided us with wonderfully positive information about our staff, its professionalism and caring. The management team has chosen to thank the staff for their much-valued work by giving them a day off of their choice.

The high point of this staff acknowledgement came when management team secretly declared one staff meeting day last summer as a 'thank you' day. After the center closed the night before our monthly meeting, the building was festively decorated, and quotes and statistics from the most recent survey were posted on every inside wall. Staff from all counties and all programs arrived early the next morning to a surprise party in their honor. The posted quotes, incidentally, remained on the walls for weeks, and garnered many interesting comments from channel members and clients. That most enjoyable day, a day when our mission was celebrated, would not have happened without the client surveys.

Our marketing efforts, like most, are ongoing. We continue to learn more about our client audience, and to formalize our mission and our marketing plan with each new bit of information.

And the proposed merger? Canceled for financial — and marketing — considerations.

Toward More Effective
Televised Anti-Drug PSAs

Denise D. Schoenbachler

SUMMARY. Historically, drug prevention public service announcement (PSA) campaigns have been ineffective in preventing drug use due to ineffective targeting and inappropriate message selection. The purpose of this paper is to address why drug prevention campaigns have failed, and to suggest ways to design more effective campaigns.

INTRODUCTION

One of the most prevalent concerns in society today is substance abuse among adolescents. Gallup polls suggest that public concern regarding this problem is increasing and that citizens believe too little is being done to deal with this growing problem (Drugs and Crime Facts 1988). Drug addiction is epidemic among adolescents with one of every six teens suffering from a severe addictive problem (Thorne and DeBlassie 1985). The statistics are frightening, especially when considering the extensive and expensive efforts made in past years to educate young people about the dangers of illicit drug use.

One prevention strategy used extensively by national and local

Denise D. Schoenbachler is affiliated with the University of Kentucky. Address correspondence to the author at: 307 B&E Building, Department of Marketing, University of Kentucky, Lexington, KY 40506.

This paper was first presented at the 1991 American Marketing Association Winter Educators' Conference. Reprinted with permission from MacKenzie, Scott and Terry Childers, Eds. (1991), *Marketing Theory and Applications* (Vol. 2) Proceedings of the American Marketing Association Winter Educators' Conference. Chicago: American Marketing Association.

organizations is the public service announcement (PSA). Like all prevention programs, PSAs have received little attention in research programs. Research efforts to aid in the development of more effective drug prevention PSAs is a social responsibility of marketers which has been ignored. The purpose of this paper is to address this responsibility through an examination of the appropriate target market and effective message appeals for drug prevention PSAs.

SETTING GOALS
FOR PSA CAMPAIGNS

PSA campaigns have usually been developed haphazardly by state or federal agencies with the goal of attracting attention. While attention is a necessary requisite of any advertising campaign, it is not enough to impact the problem of drug use. A possible goal for drug prevention campaigns is to focus on changing drug-related attitudes in order to create a negative "climate of opinion" for drug use (Donohew et al. 1989). Prevention suggests reaching the audience before drug use occurs. If a PSA campaign strives to change attitudes toward drug use, it is more likely teens' behavior will follow. A negative attitude toward drug use will be followed by behaviors consistent with this attitude and drug use will decline. Research has found that attitudes concerning the harmfulness of drug use are related to substance use behavior. A strong correlation exists between an individual's use of drugs and the attitudes and beliefs about those drugs (Sarvela and McClendon 1988). Teens tend to identify with peer groups with similar attitudes, thus a campaign which attempts to change attitudes toward drug use will help create a peer climate in which drug use is unpopular (Mosbach and Leventhal 1988). The use of PSAs is an important element in drug prevention campaigns. Television is the preeminent mass medium among adolescents and research has shown that behavioral learning does occur during television viewing (Flay and Sobel 1983). Studies have found that adolescents view the mass media as a trusted and influential source of information about drugs (Fejer and Smart 1971; Sheppard 1980). Advertising in general has been found to have both short-term and long-term effects on adolescent consumer socialization, and may act as a catalyst for interpersonal communication with family and peers (Moore and Stephens 1975; Moschis and Moore 1982).

TARGETING OF PSAs

Media only drug prevention campaigns have been largely unsuccessful in bringing about attitude or behavioral changes (Donohew et al. 1989). Part of this failure is due to the lack of focus on a specific goal, but Flay and Sobel (1983) suggest three other reasons for the failure of media prevention campaigns. First, is a lack of dissemination. PSAs are frequently aired outside of prime time or on non-commercial stations, reducing the reach and frequency of exposure (Hanneman and McEwen 1973; Flay and Sobel 1983). Second, is a lack of targeting. Many drug prevention announcements have been directed at unidentifiable audience segments. Finally, Flay and Sobel blame selectivity for the failure of PSA campaigns. Individual attitudes, values and norms affect exposure to and effectiveness of drug-related messages.

The lack of dissemination can be addressed by a well-planned approach to convince media gatekeepers of the need to air more PSAs more frequently during prime time (Flay and Sobel 1983). The problems of targeting and selectivity require much more research and attention.

The Target: Early Adolescence

If the goal of public service anti-drug campaigns is to change teens' attitude toward drug use, it is necessary to target teens who have not yet engaged in drug use behaviors, and whose attitudes toward drug use have not been formally established. Initial experimentation with most drugs usually occurs during the final three years of high school. Less than half of the heavy users of illicit drugs had begun use prior to the tenth grade (Thorne and DeBlassie 1985). The 1988 National Survey on Household Drug Abuse found 24.7% of teens age 12-17 had ever used any illicit drug.

The appropriate target for prevention PSAs is therefore early adolescents, between 11 and 14 years of age. These teens are beginning to form attitudes about drug use but most have not yet experimented heavily with drugs. To aid PSA developers in targeting early adolescents, it is necessary to identify the unique cognitive and information processing abilities of the early adolescent by reviewing the relevant developmental psychology literature.

Early adolescence is a time of dramatic change in cognitive capabilities. Inhelder and Piaget (1958) identify early adolescence as the beginning of formal operations. The major task of adolescents in this stage is the conquest of thought. The early adolescent begins to conceptualize his own thoughts and the thoughts of other people (Elkind 1981). He attempts to infer with limited accuracy the thought of others (Elkind 1985). Because of the physiological metamorphosis the young adolescent is experiencing, he is primarily concerned with himself. Because he fails to differentiate between what others are thinking about and his own thoughts, he assumes that others are as obsessed with his appearance and behavior as he is. This belief that others are preoccupied with his appearance and behavior is the crux of adolescent egocentrism (Elkind 1967).

Adolescent egocentrism, characterized by a heightened self consciousness and preoccupation with the thoughts of others, leads to the development of two constructs which further explain adolescent cognition and behavior. The first of these is the imaginary audience. Since young adolescents are so preoccupied with the thoughts of others and are equally preoccupied with their own appearance and behavior, they often anticipate the reactions of other people to themselves. Adolescents assume that others are as admiring or as critical of them as they are of themselves. The adolescent is continually constructing an imaginary audience to which he "performs" (Elkind 1967). He is always carrying within himself an imaginary peer group that is far more critical than his actual peers, who are likely to be too preoccupied with their own imaginary audience to notice others' behaviors (Newman 1985).

This imaginary peer group is very real to the early adolescent and is responsible for the intense pressure to conform to peer standards (Elkind 1989). In many respects the peer group is the single most important influence on adolescents (Elkind 1971). Some research suggests that the power of peer influence on early adolescents has increased in recent years. The amount of time parents spend with children has declined, and without substantial adult participation in directing children, they turn to peers. It is the peer group, not the family that dominates the lives of adolescents today (Dragastin and Elder 1975).

The intense pressure to conform to peer standards of behavior and attitude in early adolescence has implications for drug use as well. Adolescents have described peer group influences as global and far-reaching, affecting attitudes, values and illicit acts (O'Brien and Bierman 1988). Peer pressure has been found to be a successful predictor of drug use among adolescents (Sarvela and McClendon 1988). Membership in a peer group will be sought regardless of the price an adolescent must pay for membership. The dangers of drug use are less threatening to the early adolescent than is rejection and isolation. It is not surprising that many youngsters take drugs for one reason and one reason alone: group acceptance (Kizziar and Hagedorn 1979).

The second aspect of adolescent egocentrism which emerges with the onset of formal operations is the personal fable. The personal fable corresponds to and complements the imaginary audience. The early adolescent fails to differentiate the concerns of his own thought from those of others (imaginary audience), but at the same time, he overdifferentiates his own feelings. He feels he is of great importance to so many people, his imaginary audience, and he comes to consider himself as something special and unique (Lapsley, Milstead, and Quintana 1986). The adolescent believes only he can suffer with such intensity or experience such heightened excitement. When adolescents lament that "you don't understand how I feel," they are exemplifying the personal fable construct. The adolescent believes that his or her feelings and needs are unique, special and beyond understanding by anyone else, particularly adults (Elkind 1978). In addition, adolescents have not had time to learn the cause-effect structure of their world and often feel that the cause-effect structure does not apply to them (Newman 1985). These two factors lead the young adolescent to believe that while others will grow old and die, he will not (Elkind 1985). The personal fable leads to the adolescent's feeling of immortality and indestructibility (Lapsley 1985).

The personal fable also accounts for other bizarre adolescent behaviors. The young girl who gets pregnant despite sexual knowledge believes that others will get pregnant but not her. Her personal fable puts her above the natural order of things. Likewise, the adolescent who uses drugs, despite knowledge of the dangers, believes others will be endangered by drugs, but not him (Elkind 1978).

The imaginary audience and the personal fable dictate much of the young adolescent's cognitive thoughts, attitudes and behaviors. These two constructions account for the bizarre and often obnoxious behavior characteristic of early adolescence. They also set the young adolescent apart from childhood and adulthood. Only during this phase in development is the youngster so preoccupied with his own thoughts and the thoughts of his peers. Peer influence is at its strongest in early adolescence, affecting attitudes and behaviors. The young adolescent's perception of immortality distorts his view of the world, and leads to destructive behaviors and beliefs.

THE MESSAGE:
PHYSICAL AND SOCIAL FEAR APPEALS

Physical Fear Appeals

Having identified the target audience for PSAs as the early adolescent, appropriate messages must be used to reach this unique target. Messages designed with the characteristics of the young adolescent in mind will address the selectivity problem of PSAs identified by Flay and Sobel (1983).

PSAs often employ a "scare the hell out of them" approach (Kizziar and Hagedorn 1979). A content analysis of televised drug prevention PSAs found that over 40% depicted harmful effects of drug use (Hanneman and McEwen 1973). Research on these efforts has suggested that, as a prevention strategy, showing the extreme negative consequences of substance abuse is of marginal value (DeJong 1987).

The effectiveness of physical fear appeals in general is questionable, despite extensive research in this area. The seminal study conducted by Janis and Feshbach (1953) looked at the relationship between physical fear appeals and persuasion. They concluded that the use of a strong fear appeal, as opposed to a milder appeal, increases the likelihood that the audience will be "left in a state of emotional tension which is not fully relieved by rehearsing the reassuring recommendations contained in the communication" (p. 89). The audience is motivated to ignore or discount the threat to alleviate tension, rather than comply with the recommendations in the communications.

This research set off a series of fear appeal studies which manipulated the level of fear in a communication (Janis and Feshbach 1953; Moltz and Thistlethwaite 1955; Nunnally and Bobren 1959; Janis and Terwilliger 1962; Leventhal and Perloe 1962; Leventhal and Niles 1965; Hewgill and Miller 1965; Insko, Arkoff, and Insko 1965; Leventhal, Singer, and Jones 1965; Chu 1966; Dabbs and Leventhal 1966; Leventhal and Singer 1966; Miller and Hewgill 1966; Leventhal, Watts, and Pagano 1967; Leventhal and Trembly 1968). A review of this literature reveals considerable inconsistency among the findings. Some studies found no relationship between fear arousal and persuasion, but the methodology employed in these studies does not insure that differential fear levels were aroused in the subjects. Other studies have yielded mixed findings such as fear appeals affecting attitude change without affecting behavior change (Higbee 1969). The general conclusion emerging from the most recent research is that fear appeals do work in persuasion communication, as long as the level of fear evoked is moderate (Ray and Wilkie 1970).

Two paradigms have been proposed to explain the effectiveness of moderate versus high or low fear appeals in persuasion. The first, the fear drive paradigm, has been the predominant approach used by researchers to explain fear appeal effectiveness. The basic tenet of the fear drive paradigm is that the information contained in a message evokes an emotional reaction which then motivates a coping response. To cope with the emotion, the audience may either respond to the recommendation in the message, or discount the message (Sternthal and Craig 1974). As fear arousal increases from low to moderate levels of intensity, persuasion increases since the audience becomes more vigilant to the recommendations made in the communication. At very high levels of fear arousal, the audience becomes overly vigilant and is likely to discount the message by finding weaknesses in the position advocated, selecting nonrecommended solutions to reduce fear, or choosing some other form of denial (Janis 1967).

A second and more compelling explanation of the effects of fear arousal is posited by Leventhal (1970). Leventhal argues that the response to a fear appeal involves two parallel but independent processes. Danger control guides the audience's problem solving behavior and the action taken. The information about danger contained in the fear appeal is used by the audience to guide adaptive behavior. The second process, fear control, deals with the emotional portion of a fear appeal. Fear control guides the emotional responses of the audience. These two processes, while independent, can affect each other. If the audience response to a fear appeal is highly emotional, the fear control process inhibits the danger control process and adaptive behavior is disrupted. Likewise, adaptive behavior, guided by the danger control process, may disrupt the emotional response.

Donohew, Palmgreen, and Duncan's (1980) activation theory of information exposure has implications for fear appeal research and offers an explanation for the inverted U relationship between level of fear and effectiveness found by numerous researchers. This theory is grounded in the optimal level of arousal assumptions which suggest that people find arousal in moderate amounts to be pleasurable. Each individual has a unique optimal level of arousal, below which he is bored and above which he is over stimulated (Donohew et al. 1989). When applied to fear appeal messages, the activation theory suggests that mild appeals are below the optimal level of arousal and are virtually ignored. At a moderate level, arousal is optimal, the audience attends, and attitude and behavior changes are likely. Very high fear levels are above the optimal arousal and the audience is likely to turn away or discount the communication.

Finally, Rogers (1975) extended Leventhal's parallel process paradigm to form a protection motivation theory. Based on the premise that cognitive processes are more important than emotional processes in mediating attitude change, Rogers turned to expectancy-value theory to explain the effectiveness of fear appeals. Expectancy-value theory suggests that the tendency to perform a behavior is a function of the expectancy that the behavior will be followed by certain consequences and the value of those consequences. When exposed to a fear communication, the audience appraises the severity of the depicted event, estimates the probability of occurrence of the event, and assesses its belief in the efficacy of the recommended coping response.

Rogers' protection motivation theory helps explain the inconsistent findings of fear appeal research. Most research prior to Rogers examined only one of the three variables identified, magnitude of noxiousness or level of fear. In other research, probability of occurrence or efficacy of the recommended coping response were measured, but the combination and interaction effects of the three variables were not controlled. Rogers' theory addresses the nonmonotonic relationships between fear appeals and attitude or behavior change identified by Janis and other fear appeal researchers. He argues that the studies which found such relationships did not account for all three variables in fear appeals. According to Rogers, the relationship between fear arousal and attitude and behavior change can take on many shapes, depending on the variation of the three variables he suggests are key to understanding fear appeal effectiveness (Rogers 1975).

Social Fear Appeals

The theories presented which attempt to explain the effectiveness of fear appeals have focused on only one type of fear appeal, the physically threatening fear appeal. Absent from this discussion has been the socially threatening fear appeal. The physical fear appeal is defined as fear of personal bodily harm. Social fear is the threat of social disapproval by significant others (Unger and Stearns 1984). Whether the findings and theories of physical fear appeals can be applied to social fear appeals is questionable. Fear researchers have virtually ignored the effects of the social fear appeal. The effect of threatening social consequences has been examined in only one study (Sternthal and Craig 1974). This study did reveal that both social approval and social disapproval were more effective in changing attitudes towards blood donation to the Red Cross than were messages that implied no consequences. Social disapproval was substantially more effective in changing attitudes than was social approval. The results of one study cannot be generalized to conclude that social disapproval is more effective than social approval, yet this study has implications for future research examining social fear appeals.

Perhaps the most obvious question looming is whether social fear appeals and physical fear appeals are equally effective. No study has attempted to compare the effectiveness of these two appeals. Furthermore, interaction effects of level of fear and social appeals has yet to be examined (Unger and Stearns 1984).

TOWARD MORE EFFECTIVE PSA CAMPAIGNS

In order to produce effective PSA campaigns, goal setting, targeting and message construction must be considered holistically. It is not enough to concentrate on one of these key factors; all three must work harmoniously to effectively impact substance abuse among adolescents. As suggested, the appropriate goal for PSA campaigns is to change attitudes in order to create an unfavorable climate of opinion about drugs among teens. To create a global, negative attitude towards drug use, it is imperative that PSA campaigns be targeted at the young adolescent, who has not yet formed a definitive attitude towards drug use and who is not currently a heavy drug user. If the characteristics of the early adolescent and the features of fear appeals are combined, effective PSA campaigns can be formulated to deal with the problem of drug abuse.

Two characteristics of the early adolescent have been identified which will impact the effectiveness of a fear appeal PSA. First, is the personal fable. The adolescent believes he is immortal and carries an "it will never happen to me" belief which guides his cognitive and information processing abilities. If the adolescent believes he is immortal, it is ludicrous to consider a physically threatening fear appeal message. The cognitive response of the early adolescent to such a message is one of discounting the probability of occurrence.

The second feature of the targeted early adolescent implies the appropriate message appeal. The imaginary audience aspect of the adolescent suggests that his attitudes and behaviors are directed towards an imaginary peer group. The imaginary audience is a reflection of the teen's peer group, and the teen strictly conforms to the attitudes, beliefs and accepted behaviors of the peer group. Clearly, if the attitude of the peer group is anti-drug, members of the group and teens aspiring to belong to the group will adopt anti-drug attitudes to conform.

Although limited, the research on socially threatening fear appeals suggests that this appeal is the answer for PSA campaigns aimed at early adolescents. Social disapproval messages have been found to be effective at influencing attitude change, and would be particularly effective for the early adolescent who is constantly striving for social approval. PSAs which connect social disapproval with drug use will elicit a response via the imaginary audience. A social disapproval message would be extremely effective if it depicted teens disapproving of the attitudes and behaviors of other teen drug users. This type of message would, in effect, create an imaginary audience for which adolescent viewers would perform.

The interacting aspect of level of fear with type of fear will impact the effectiveness of the PSA campaign aimed at adolescents. Research suggests moderate levels of fear are most effective when the goal is attitude change. In the case of a socially threatening fear appeal, this will hold true. Because of the perceived noxiousness of social disapproval, a high level of fear may activate the danger control process or be above the optimal level of arousal, reducing the effectiveness of the message. Low levels of fear may not activate the imaginary audience and will therefore be less effective.

In the case of physically threatening fear appeals, level of fear is a less important factor since this type of appeal is less effective than the socially threatening fear appeal. It is possible, however, that very high levels of physical fear depiction will overide the personal fable and be somewhat influential in affecting attitudes towards drug use. When the early adolescent is the target, the level of fear in a physically threatening fear appeal will be positively related to effectiveness. Low and moderate fear appeals will be discounted via the personal fable. At very high levels, the adolescent may begin to question the value of the personal fable and attitude change is possible. This positive relationship between level of physical fear and effectiveness is supported by activation theory. While each individual has a unique optimal level of arousal, it has been suggested that this level may be higher for adolescents (Zuckerman 1978). Adolescents may need greater stimulation to be aroused, and are therefore able to accept higher levels of arousal such as those found in high levels of physically threatening fear appeals.

The preceding discussion of early adolescence and fear appeal effectiveness, derived from developmental psychology and fear appeal research, suggests several propositions worthy of consideration by researchers:

Proposition 1: Socially threatening, social disapproval appeals will be more effective than physically threatening fear appeals in changing attitudes towards drug use in young adolescents.

Proposition 2: There is an inverted U-shape relationship between level of fear and effectiveness in changing attitudes toward drug use when a socially threatening fear appeal is used.

Proposition 3: There is a positive relationship between level of fear and effectiveness in changing attitudes toward drug use when a physically threatening fear appeal is used.

Proposition 4: Depicting adolescents as spokespersons in PSAs will increase the effectiveness of drug prevention fear appeals.

PSA campaigns will achieve the goal of global anti-drug attitudes among adolescents only if they acknowledge the appropriate target and message. This paper suggests that the early adolescent is the appropriate target to impact drug use attitudes in the long run. To reach this audience, PSAs must change their appeal. Physically threatening fear appeals are not the optimal choice for this target. Only moderate levels of socially threatening fear appeals will effectively impact the attitudes of the early adolescent. Research has determined the importance of social approval and conformity to peer attitudes among adolescents. It has also suggested that the belief system of adolescents includes an element of immortality. PSA campaigns must acknowledge these facts when designing messages to reach the early adolescent when the goal of the campaign is global attitude change.

REFERENCES

Chu, Godwin C. (1966), "Fear Arousal, Efficacy, and Imminency," *Journal of Personality and Social Psychology*, 4 (5), 517-524.

Dabbs, James M. Jr., and Howard Leventhal (1966), "Effects of Varying the Recommendations in a Fear-Arousing Communication," *Journal of Personality and Social Psychology*, 4 (5), 525-531.

DeJong, William (1987), "A Short-term Evaluation of Project Dare (Drug Abuse Resistance Education): Preliminary Indications of Effectiveness," *Journal of Drug Education*, 17 (4), 279-294.

Donohew, Lewis, Philip Palmgreen, and J. Duncan (1980), "An Activation Model of Information Exposure," *Communication Monographs*, 47, 295-303.

––––––, Philip Palmgreen, Elizabeth Lorch, Mary Rogus, David Helm and Nancy Grant (1989), "Sensation Seeking and Targeting of Televised Anti-Drug PSAs," paper presented at the Annual Conference of the International Communication Association, San Francisco, CA.

Dragastin, Sigmund E. and Glen H. Elder, Jr. (1975), *Adolescence in the Life Cycle: Psychological Change and Social Context,* Washington, DC: Hemisphere Publishing.

Drugs and Crime Facts (1988), Washington, DC: Government Printing Office.

Elkind, David (1967), "Egocentrism in Adolescence," *Child Development,* 38, 1025-1034.

–––––– (1971), *A Sympathetic Understanding of the Child Six to Sixteen,* Boston, MA: Oxford University Press.

–––––– (1978), "Understanding the Young Adolescent," *Adolescence,* 13 (Spring), 127-134.

–––––– (1981) *Children and Adolescents*, New York, NY: Random House, Inc.

–––––– (1985), "Cognitive Development and Adolescent Disabilities," *Journal of Adolescent Health Care*, 6, 84-89.

–––––– (1989), "What Happens when Markers of Maturity Disappear?" *The Education Digest*, 54 (January), 34-36.

Fejer, D. and R. Smart (1971), "Sources of Information about Drugs Among High School Students," *Public Opinion Quarterly,* 35 (2), 235-241.

Flay, B.R and J.L. Sobel (1983), "The Role of Mass Media in Preventing Adolescent Substance Abuse," in *Preventing Adolescent Drug Abuse: Intervention Strategies,* eds. T.J. Glynn et al., NIDA Research Monograph Series (47).

Hanneman, Gerhard J. and William J. McEwen (1973), "Televised Drug Abuse Appeals: A Content Analysis," *Journalism Quarterly,* 50 (2), 329-333.

Hewgill, Murray A. and Gerald R. Miller (1965), "Source Credibility and Response to Fear-Arousing Communications," *Speech Monographs,* 32 (June), 95-101.

Higbee, Kenneth L. (1969), "Fifteen Years of Fear Arousal: Research on Threat Appeals: 1953-1968," *Psychological Bulletin,* 72 (6), 426-444.

Inhelder, B. and Jean Piaget (1958), *The Growth of Logical Thinking from Childhood to Adolescence,* New York, NY: Basic Books.

Insko, C.A., A. Arkoff, and V.M. Insko (1965), "Effects of High and Low Fear-arousing Communications upon Opinions Toward Smoking," *Journal of Experimental Social Psychology,* 1 (August), 256-266.

Janis, Irving L. (1967), "Effects of Fear Arousal on Attitude Change: Recent Developments in Theory and Experimental Research," *Advances in Experimental Social Psychology,* 3, 167-225.

_____ and Seymour Feshbach (1953), "Effects of Fear-Arousing Communications," *Journal of Abnormal and Social Psychology,* 48 (1), 78-92.

_____ and Robert F. Terwilliger (1962), "An Experimental Study of Psychological Resistances to Fear Arousing Communications," *Journal of Abnormal and Social Psychology,* 65 (6), 403-410.

Kizziar, Janet W. and Judy Hagedorn (1979), *Search for Acceptance: The Adolescent and Self-Esteem,* Chicago, IL: Nelson-Hall.

Lapsley, Daniel K. (1985), "Elkind on Egocentrism," *Developmental Review,* 5, 227-236.

_____, Matt Milstead, and Stephen M. Quintana (1986), "Adolescent Egocentrism and Formal Operations: Tests of a Theoretical Assumption," *Developmental Psychology,* 22 (6), 800-807.

Leventhal, Howard (1970), "Findings and Theory in the Study of Fear Communications," in *Advances in Experimental Social Psychology,* Vol. 5, ed. L. Berkowitz, New York: Academic Press, 119-186.

_____ and P. Niles (1965), "Persistence of Influence for Varying Durations of Exposure to Threat Stimuli," *Psychological Reports,* 16, 223-233.

_____ and S. Perloe (1962), "A Relationship Between Self-esteem and Persuasibility," *Journal of Abnormal and Social Psychology,* 64, 385-388.

_____ and Robert Singer (1966), "Affect Arousal and Positioning of Recommendations in Persuasive Communications," *Journal of Personality and Social Psychology,* 4, 137-146.

_____, Robert Singer, and Susan Jones (1965), "Effects of Fear and Specificity of Recommendation upon Attitudes and Behavior," *Journal of Personality and Social Psychology,* 2 (1), 20-29.

_____ and G. Trembly (1968), "Negative Emotions and Persuasion," *Journal of Personality,* 36, 154-168.

_____, Jean C. Watts, and Francia Pagano (1967), "Effects of Fear and Instructions on How to Cope with Danger," *Journal of Personality and Social Psychology,* 6 (3), 313-321.

Miller, Gerald R. and Murray A. Hewgill (1966), "Some Recent Research on Fear-arousing Message Appeals," *Speech Monographs,* 33 (4), 377-391.

Moltz, H. and Donald L. Thistlethwaite (1955), "Attitude Modification and Anxiety Reduction," *Journal of Abnormal and Social Psychology,* 9, 251-256.

Moore, Roy L. and Lowndes F. Stephens (1975), "Some Communication and Demographic Determinants of Adolescent Consumer Learning," *Journal of Consumer Research,* 2 (September), 80-92.

Mosbach, Peter and Howard Leventhal (1988), "Peer Group Identification and Smoking: Implications for Intervention," *Journal of Abnormal Psychology,* 97 (2), 238-245.

Moschis, George P. and Roy L. Moore (1982), "A Longitudinal Study of Television Advertising Effects," *Journal of Consumer Research,* 9 (December), 279-287.

National Household Survey on Drug Abuse (1988), U.S. Department of Health and Human Services, 17.

Newman, Joan (1985), "Adolescents: Why They Can Be So Obnoxious," *Adolescence,* 20 (Fall), 635-645.

Nunnally, J.C. and H. Bobren (1959), "Variables Governing the Willingness to Receive Communications on Mental Health," *Journal of Personality,* 27, 38-46.

O'Brien, Susan F. and Karen Linn Bierman (1988), "Conceptions and Perceived Influence of Peer Groups: Interviews with Preadolescents and Adolescents," *Child Development,* 59, 1360-1365.

Ray, Michael L. and William L. Wilkie (1970), "Fear: The Potential of an Appeal Neglected by Marketing," *Journal of Marketing,* 34 (January), 54-62.

Rogers, Ronald W. (1975), "A Protection Motivation Theory of Fear Appeals and Attitude Change," *The Journal of Psychology,* 91, 93-114.

Sarvela, Paul D. and E.J. McClendon (1988), "Indicators of Rural Youth Drug Use," *Journal of Youth and Adolescence,* 17 (4), 335-347.

Sheppard, M.A. (1980), "Sources of Information about Drugs," *Journal of Drug Education,* 10 (3), 257-262.

Sternthal, Brian and C. Samuel Craig (1974), "Fear Appeals: Revisited and Revised," *Journal of Consumer Research,* 1 (December), 22-34.

Thorne, Craig R. and Richard R. DeBlassie (1985), "Adolescent Substance Abuse," *Adolescence,* 20 (Summer), 335-347.

Unger, Lynette S. and James M. Stearns (1984), "The Use of Fear and Guilt Messages in Television Advertising: Issues and Evidence," in *Advances in Consumer Research,* Vol. 11, ed. Thomas C. Kinnear, Provo, UT: Association for Consumer Research, 16-20.

Zuckerman, Marvin (1978), "The Search for High Sensation," *Psychology Today,* (February), 38-40; 43; 46; 96; 99.

The Dissemination and Content of Drug Prevention Public Service Announcements

Denise D. Schoenbachler
Margaret U. Dsilva

SUMMARY. Drug prevention public service announcement (PSA) campaigns have historically been unsuccessful, in part because of dissemination problems and a lack of targeting and message development. This study looked at one week's television programming to address the dissemination issue. Content analysis was used to discern the target and type of appeals used in drug prevention PSAs. Implications for future research to aid PSA developers in creating effective PSAs are discussed.

INTRODUCTION

Televised anti-drug public service announcements (PSAs) represent a part of the nationwide campaign to address the problem of drug abuse among teens. While PSAs have been produced and disseminated for several decades, media-only drug prevention campaigns have been largely unsuccessful in bringing about change because they have failed to reach their target audience (Capalaces and Starr 1973; Hanneman 1973; Hu and Mitchell 1978; Delaney 1978). Despite the poor record of drug prevention PSAs, researchers have failed to examine the content of drug prevention PSAs to discern why they have failed. A content analysis of drug prevention

---

Denise D. Schoenbachler is affiliated with the University of Kentucky, Department of Marketing, 307 B&E Building, Lexington, KY 40506. Margaret U. Dsilva is affiliated with the University of Kentucky, Department of Communications, 227 Grehan Building, Lexington, KY 40506.
The authors wish to thank Dr. Tommy E. Whittler and Dr. Phillip Palmgreen for their helpful comments.

179

PSAs would also establish a base for future research which examines the elements necessary to strengthen the media component of drug prevention efforts. The purpose of this paper therefore, is to examine the dissemination and analyze the content of drug prevention PSAs.

BACKGROUND

Flay and Sobel (1983) suggest that drug prevention PSAs have historically been unsuccessful because they have not been widely disseminated. PSAs are often aired outside of prime time or on noncommercial stations, reducing the reach and frequency of exposure (Brown & Einsiedel 1990). Hanneman and McEwen (1973) addressed the issue of dissemination in the most recent content analysis of PSAs and found only about 6% of drug prevention PSAs aired during prime time. Using Hanneman and McEwen's work as a baseline, this study seeks to determine if there has been a move toward more frequent, prime time airing of drug prevention PSAs.

A lack of targeting represents another failure of drug prevention PSAs (Flay and Sobel 1983; Solomon 1989; Atkin and Freimuth 1989; Donohew 1990). Most PSAs are developed with little formative research to determine the appropriate target and how to reach that target (Atkin and Freimuth 1989; Rogers and Storey 1987). In the 1973 content analysis (Hanneman and McEwen 1973), 49% of the PSAs coded were targeted to a "general" audience. Only about 18% were targeted toward youth, and 33% toward parents. Thus, close to half of the PSAs had no discernible target audience. The present content analysis evaluates the extent to which the concept of targeting has been adopted by PSA producers. Can a target be identified, and if so, what is the target audience for drug prevention PSAs?

Drug prevention PSA campaigns have historically followed the prevailing public health campaign genre in terms of message appeals. Typically, only minimal background information about the target audience is used in designing message appeals, and the normative standards of health campaign messages prevail. "Messages tend to be produced in a haphazard fashion based on the whim of copywriters or artists" (Atkin and Freimuth 1989).

The prevailing health campaign appeal has focused on scaring viewers into attitude or behavior changes through the use of physical and social fear appeals (Kizziar and Hagedorn 1979; King and Reid 1990). Hanneman and McEwen (1973) found 20% of the PSAs emphasized physical effects of drug use and 22% concentrated on the social effects. The remaining PSAs used a celebrity appeal or presented factual information about drug use. Similarly, Reid and King found physical fear appeals the dominant approach used in drinking and driving PSAs (1986).

The effectiveness of fear appeals is questionable, despite extensive research in this area. The findings in fear appeal studies have been mixed; with some suggesting fear appeals are effective, others suggest not. The optimal level of fear in an appeal has varied from very low to very high, depending on the study reviewed, although the preponderance of evidence suggests a moderate level of fear is most effective (Higbee 1969; Ray and Wilkie 1970; Sternthal and Craig 1974).

The use of fear appeals in public communication campaigns has received little attention, but the work done in this area suggests that fear appeals may not be effective in bringing about attitude or behavior change (King and Reid 1990; DeJong 1987; Ray and Ward 1976; Feingold and Knapp 1977). Given this preliminary evidence, drug prevention PSAs should be starting to rely on other types of message appeals. This study addresses the issue of the use of various appeals in drug prevention PSAs by examining the extent to which physical and social fear appeals are currently used, and what alternative appeals are used in PSAs. Previous research suggests that a moderate level of fear is preferable, yet PSAs have historically used high levels of fear. If fear appeals are still found in drug prevention PSAs, this study evaluates the level of fear employed in these appeals.

THE STUDY

Method

To obtain a set of drug prevention PSAs for content analysis, the three major television networks, ABC, NBC and CBS, were videotaped for seven consecutive days from July 31, 1990 to August 6, 1990, from 9 a.m. until 11 p.m. in a medium sized Southeastern city serving a market of approximately 1 million viewers. A total of 274 hours of programming was recorded, then reviewed to pull out the drug prevention PSAs. The station, time, date and program airing were recorded for each viewing of a PSA. The PSAs were then copied to another tape for coding later. A total of 13 different PSAs, shown a total of 19 times, were found during the sample time period.

Five adult coders independently viewed and analyzed the complete set of PSAs using specified categories of analysis on a coding sheet. The objective in this study was not to develop expert judges, therefore minimal training of coders was conducted.

Because many of the drug prevention PSAs are directed at adolescents, five coders age 14-15 were also employed to evaluate the content of the PSAs. The coding results of the two groups were compared and no differences found. Therefore, the combined coding results for the two groups were used to evaluate the content of drug prevention PSAs.

Categories of Analysis

The categories of analysis used for the coding of content included the target of the ad, the primary appeal of the ad, and the level of fear apparent in the ad. These categories reflect the criticisms of drug prevention PSAs addressed by Flay and Sobel (1983), as well as the criticism of the use of fear in drug prevention messages (De-Jong 1987).

The target of the ad was coded using a 5 point forced choice scale, including no target, parents, youth, adults or other. The appeal category also was a 5 point forced choice scale. The choices included: (1) "creates fear of bodily harm" (2) "creates fear of being socially isolated" (3) "uses the appeal of a celebrity" (4) "gives factual information" (5) "identifies alternatives to drugs." The level of fear was measured using a 7 point scale from 1-no fear to 7-high fear in response to the question, "how much fear (threat of bodily harm or social isolation) do you think was apparent in the ad?"

Intercoder agreement was assessed for the two coder groups individually and for the combined group. Holsti's (1969) composite reliability score for greater than two coders was used, and adjusted for chance agreement using Scott's pi (1955). Table 1 presents the Scott's pi index of reliability for the individual coder groups and for the combined group for each of the three major categories.

The reliability indices range from .81 for the adult coding of level of fear to .95 for the combined coding for target. All of the reliability indices are in the acceptable range according to Kassarjian (1977).

RESULTS

Dissemination

The issue of the dissemination of drug prevention PSAs identified by Flay and Sobel (1983) can be examined by looking at the

TABLE 1

Inter-Coder Agreement and Reliability

Content items	Inter-Coder Agreement (a)	Inter-Coder Reliability (b)
Target		
Adults	.95	.92
Teens	.94	.91
Combined	.97	.95
Type of Appeal		
Adults	.91	.87
Teens	.93	.89
Combined	.96	.93
Level of Fear		
Adults	.85	.81
Teens	.86	.82
Combined	.88	.85

(a) Holsti's composite agreement
(b) Scott's pi index of reliability

frequency, programming context and times shown of PSAs. The limited number of PSAs shown during the sample period suggests that media gatekeepers are reluctant to provide the air time for frequent showing of PSAs. Only thirteen different PSAs were aired a total of nineteen times.

While PSAs are shown relatively infrequently, it appears that these ads are being aired more in prime time. Hanneman and McEwen (1973) found that only 6% of drug prevention PSAs were aired during prime time. Table 2 shows that the current study found 53% shown from 8-11 p.m. Forty-two percent were aired from 9 a.m. until 3 p.m., and only 5% from 3-8 p.m.

Media gatekeepers are providing valuable air time, although in limited quantities, to the PSAs. Table 3 describes the programming context in which the ads were aired.

Most of the PSAs were aired during highly rated programs for both youths and parents. In every viewing night in the sample, at least one drug prevention PSA was aired during prime time. A second popular time spot for youths, Saturday morning, contained about 20% of the PSA airings.

It is difficult to generalize the dissemination results for PSAs to other regions since the decision to air PSAs is done primarily at the local station affiliation level. In the sample market, 63% of the PSAs were aired on ABC, 21% on NBC and 16% on CBS. All of the PSAs shown during the time period are likely to be available for

TABLE 2

DISSEMINATION OF PSAs

Time Aired	Number of PSAs	Percentage of PSAs
9am-3pm	8	42%
3pm-8pm	1	5%
8pm-11pm	10	53%

TABLE 3

PSA TARGET, TIME SHOWN, AND PROGRAM CONTEXT

PSAs TARGETED AT YOUTH

Time Shown	Program Context
9:50am	Ninth & O Baptist Church
10:20am	Life Choices
10:30am	House Party
12:00noon	Bugs Bunny and Friends
8:20pm	Murder, She Wrote
8:20pm	MacGyver
8:20pm	Major Dad
8:30pm	Wonder Years
8:50pm	Monopoly
9:50pm	Anything But Love

PSAs TARGETED AT PARENTS

9:15am	Captain N: The Game Master
9:20am	Regis and Kathy Lee
2:00pm	All My Children
8:15pm	13 East
8:30pm	Father Dowling Mysteries

PSAs HAVING NO TARGET

10:30am	Ghostbusters
7:30pm	Life Goes On
8:15pm	Prime Time Pets

airing in numerous television markets since all were produced by national organizations. Eleven of the PSAs were produced by Partnership for a Drug-Free America, one by the California Governor's Council, and one by the US Army Reserve. Generally, these professionally produced, national PSAs are sent to most television affiliates for airing.

Targeting

While Flay and Sobel (1983) suggest most PSAs are directed at unidentifiable targets, the current study found high inter-coder agreement on identification of the target of the PSAs examined. Fifty-four percent of the ads were directed toward youths, 31% at parents, and only 15% were identified as having no target. Table 3 identifies the target of the PSAs and the program context in which they were aired. The programming context in which an ad appears influences the effectiveness of the advertisement (Schumann and Thorson 1990). Krugman (1987) hypothesized that due to a "spillover" effect, commercials may be more effective when placed in well-liked programs.

Table 3 suggests that not only do PSAs have identifiable targets, but are shown in appropriate contexts given the target. Sixty-four percent of the PSAs aimed at youths were shown during prime time, a heavy viewing time for this target. Nine percent were shown Saturday morning, and the remaining 27% were aired in the morning between 9-11 a.m. The 27% aired during morning hours may be considered "off times" but the sample time frame was in the summer months when youths are home during the day. The reach of these ads may, therefore, be greater than expected.

Of the 31% of the PSAs directed toward parents, 40% were aired during prime time, 40% during adult-target daytime programs and 20% on Saturday morning. Thus, 80% of these parent-targeted PSAs were aired during programs likely to be watched by parents. The Saturday morning time is primarily a youth market, but parents may be watching these programs with youths and view the PSAs.

Only three of the PSAs (15%) aired during the week were coded as "no target." Of these, 67% were shown during prime time, and

33% on Saturday morning. With no identifiable target, it is impossible to discern if these PSAs would reach youths or parents.

Type of Appeal

Despite the questionable effectiveness of physical fear appeals in PSAs, 62% of the ads in the sample were coded as using primarily a physical threat appeal (see Table 4).

The celebrity appeal was the second most popular approach and 15% of the ads coded used this type of appeal. Social threat appeals and identifying alternatives to drugs were both evident in only 8% of the ads, and presentation of factual information in 7%.

Comparing these results to those of Hanneman and McEwen (1973) suggests that the use of physical threats is increasing, while the presentation of factual information is decreasing. Hanneman and McEwen found only 20% of their sample ads using physical threats, 22% used social threats, and 21% presented factual information. This comparison suggests that PSA producers continue to follow the prevailing health campaign genre; use of physical threats.

All of the PSAs produced by Partnership for a Drug-free America used either a social or physical threat. These messages are professionally produced and widely disseminated yet seem to ignore the

TABLE 4

TYPE OF APPEAL USED IN PSAs

Type of Appeal	Number of PSAs	Percentage
Physical Fear Appeal	8	62%
Social Fear Appeal	1	8%
Celebrity Appeal	2	15%
Identifies Alternatives to Drugs	1	8%
Presented Factual Information	1	7%

evidence suggesting fear appeals may not be the most effective approach in PSA campaigns (King and Reid 1990).

Level of Fear

The majority of fear appeal research suggests that a moderate or low level of fear is most effective. The PSAs viewed in this sample used primarily high levels of fear (see Table 5).

Almost half (46%) scored a 6 or 7 on the 7 point scale, suggesting high levels of fear. Almost 16% used a medium level, and 23% low levels of fear. About 16% of the ads received mixed coding results when the adult and teen coders were combined. The teen coders coded two ads as high fear (score of 6), while the adult coders gave the same ads the lowest score of 1. This discrepancy raises the question of what exactly is threatening to teens versus adults. It is possible that different threats in messages lead to differing levels of fear arousal in teens than in adults.

DISCUSSION

The purpose of content analyzing drug prevention PSAs was to ascertain the current quantitative and qualitative aspects of these messages. The information produced in this study provides direc-

TABLE 5

LEVEL OF FEAR PRESENT IN PSAs

Level of Fear	Percentage
High Fear (Score of 6 or 7)	46.0%
Medium Fear (Score of 3-5)	15.5%
Low Fear (Score of 1 or 2)	23.0%
Mixed Results	15.5%

tion for future research and identifies problem areas in PSA media campaigns.

While the dissemination of PSAs has improved over the past 17 years in terms of time of airing, the frequency of airing remains minimal. There is still a need to convince media gatekeepers of the importance of frequent airing of drug prevention PSAs. Television is the preeminent mass medium among adolescents and research has shown that behavioral learning does occur during television viewing (Flay and Sobel 1983). Adolescents view the mass media as a trusted and influential source of information about drugs (Fejer and Smart 1971; Sheppard 1980). It is therefore necessary for more frequent, prime time airing of PSAs to insure that adolescents receive appropriate information about drugs. While it is difficult to envision media producers giving up valuable advertising time, perhaps organizations can be convinced of the value of buying time to air PSAs. One airing of a PSA found in this study was paid for by Procter & Gamble, illustrating the opportunity for organizations to increase their image as socially responsible and provide a valuable public service as well. Perhaps PSA producers should focus their dissemination efforts on organizations paying for PSA airings, rather than on convincing media gatekeepers to provide "free" airing time.

This study found that PSAs are identifying targets and attempting to reach these targets through appropriate program context. Most PSAs are aimed at youth, but unfortunately adolescents have been virtually ignored in advertising and drug abuse literature (Sarvela and McClendon 1988). Thus, PSA developers are left with no guidelines for creating messages to reach this audience. This lack of research support for PSA development explains the continued dependence on the prevailing health campaign genre; fear appeals. Most of the PSAs found in this study used high levels of physical fear despite conflicting evidence on the use of fear appeals.

This extensive use of fear appeals in drug prevention PSAs suggests the need for an examination of the effectiveness of fear appeals on youth in a drug prevention context. Future research needs to establish the effectiveness of levels of fear on attitudes toward drug use and behavioral intention to use drugs. Current studies have used subjects in the 18-21 age range. Future research should focus on younger adolescents whose attitudes toward drugs may not be as firmly established. Finally, the use of social fear appeals in drug prevention PSAs has declined since Hanneman and McEwen's research. Research on social fear appeals is generally lacking in the literature, but should be examined in a drug prevention context. Youth, the target of most PSAs, are very concerned with peer approval and may respond more favorably to messages suggesting disapproval of drug use (Elkind 1989).

This study has identified some of the key problems in the dissemination of drug prevention PSAs and has established a base line for future research on developing more effective drug prevention PSAs. The importance of this issue cannot be overstated. Drug use among adolescents is a critical problem in our society. If prevention programs continue to rely heavily on the media through the use of PSAs, it is necessary for marketing and advertising researchers to provide PSA developers with information to aid in creating effective PSAs.

REFERENCES

Atkin, Charles K. and Vicki Freimuth (1989), "Formative Evaluation Research in Campaign Design," in *Public Communication Campaigns,* Ronald E. Rice and Charles K. Atkin, eds., Newbury Park, CA: SAGE Publications, Inc., 131-150.

Brown, Jane D. and Edna F. Einsiedel (1990), "Public Health Campaigns: Mass Media Strategies," in *Communication and Health*, Eileen Berlin Ray and Lewis Donohew, eds., Hillsdale, NJ: Lawrence Erlbaum Associates, Inc., 153-170.

Capalaces, Roger and J. Starr (1973), "The Negative Message of Anti-drug Spots: Does it get Across?" *Public Telecommunications Review* (1), 64-66.

DeJong, William (1987), "A Short-term Evaluation of Project Dare (Drug Abuse Resistance Education): Preliminary Indications of Effectiveness," *Journal of Drug Education*, 17 (4), 279-294.

Delaney, Robert W. (1978), Comparison Impact of Two Approaches to Primary Alcoholism Prevention in Florida—1978, Sarasota, Florida: Department of Health and Rehabilitative Services, Alcohol Abuse Prevention Project.

Donohew, Lewis (1990), "Public Health Campaigns: Individual Message Strategies," in *Communication and Health,* Eileen Berlin Ray and Lewis Donohew, eds., Hillsdale, NJ: Lawrence Erlbaum Associates, 136-152.

Elkind, David (1989), "What Happens when Markers of Maturity Disappear?" *The Education Digest*, 54 (January), 34-36.

Feingold, Paul C. and Mark L. Knapp (1977), "Anti-Drug Abuse Commercials," *Journal of Communications,* 27 (Winter), 20-28.

Fejer, D. and Smart, R. (1971), "Sources of Information about Drugs Among High School Students," *Public Opinion Quarterly,* 35 (2), 235-241.

Flay, Brian R. and Judith L. Sobel (1983), "The Role of Mass Media in Preventing Adolescent Substance Abuse," in *Preventing Adolescent Drug Abuse: Intervention Strategies,* Thomas J. Glynn, Carl G. Leukefeld, and Jacqueline P. Ludford, eds., NIDA Research Monograph 47, 5-35.

Hanneman, Gerhard J. (1973), "Communicating Drug Abuse Information Among College Students," *Public Opinion Quarterly,* 37 (2), 171-191.

Hanneman, Gerhard J. and William J. McEwen (1973), "Televised Drug Abuse Appeals: a Content Analysis," *Journalism Quarterly,* 50 (2), 329-333.

Higbee, Kenneth L. (1969), "Fifteen Years of Fear Arousal: Research on Threat Appeals: 1953-1968," *Psychological Bulletin,* 72 (6), 426-444.

Holsti, Ole R. (1969), *Content Analysis for the Social Sciences and Humanities,* Reading, Mass.: Addison-Wesley Publishing Co.

Hu, T. and M. Mitchell (1978), Cost Effectiveness Evaluation of the 1978 Media Drug Abuse Prevention Television Campaign, A final report submitted to the Prevention Branch, National Institute on Drug Abuse.

Kassarjian, Harold (1977), "Content Analysis in Consumer Research," *Journal of Consumer Research,* 4 (June), 8-18.

King, Karen Whitehill and Leonard N. Reid (1990), "Fear Arousing Anti-Drinking and Driving PSAs: Do Physical Injury Threats Influence Young Adults?" in *Current Issues and Research in Advertising,* James H. Leigh and Claude R. Martin, Jr. eds., Ann Arbor, MI: The University of Michigan.

Kizziar, Janet W. and Judy Hagedorn (1979), *Search for Acceptance: The Adolescent and Self-esteem,* Chicago, IL: Nelson-Hall.

Krugman, Dean (1987), "The Television Viewing Environment: Implications of Audience Change," Paper presented to Cable TV Advertising: In Search of the Right Formula, Columbia University, New York, May 8.

Ray, Michael and Scott Ward (1976), "Experimentation for Pretesting Public Health Campaigns," in *Advances in Consumer Research,* Association for Consumer Research, 3, 278-286.

———, and William Wilkie (1970), "Fear: The Potential of an Appeal Neglected by Marketing," *Journal of Marketing,* 34 (January), 54-62.

Reid, Leonard N. and Karen Whitehill King (1986), "The Characteristics of Anti-Drinking and Driving PSAs: A Preliminary Look," in *Proceedings of the 1986 Conference of the American Academy of Advertising,* Earnest F. Larkin, ed., Norman, OK: University of Oklahoma, 103-106.

Rogers, Everett M. and J. Douglas Storey (1987), "Communication Campaigns," in *Handbook of Communication Science,* Charles R. Berger and Steven H. Chaffee, eds., Newbury Park, CA: SAGE Publications.

Sarvela, Paul D. and E.J. McClendon (1988), "Indicators of Rural Youth Drug Use," *Journal of Youth and Adolescence,* 17 (4), 335-347.

Schumann, David W. and Esther Thorson (1990), "The Influence of Viewing

Context on Commercial Effectiveness: A Selection-Processing Model,'' in *Current Issues and Research in Advertising,* James H. Leigh and Claude R. Martin, Jr., eds., Ann Arbor, MI: The University of Michigan.

Scott, William A. (1955), ''Reliability of Content Analysis: The Case of Nominal Scale Coding,'' *Public Opinion Quarterly*, 19, 321-325.

Sheppard, M.A. (1980), ''Sources of Information about Drugs,'' *Journal of Drug Education*, 10 (3), 257-262.

Solomon, Douglas S. (1989), ''A Social Marketing Perspective on Communication Campaigns,'' in *Public Communication Campaigns*, Ronald E. Rice and Charles K. Atkin, eds., Newbury Park, CA: SAGE Publications, Inc.

Sternthal, Brian and C. Samuel Craig (1974), ''Fear Appeals: Revisited and Revised,'' *Journal of Consumer Research*, 1 (December), 22-34.

Reports from the Field:
Marketing Success:
A Case Study of NAMI's Growing
Visibility and Outreach

Charles R. Harman

INTRODUCTION

I read about your organization in READER'S DIGEST and was hoping that you could help me. My 40 year old son who lives with me suffers from schizophrenia. He hears voices, lives in isolation, but doesn't believe anything is wrong with him. Our family has gone through hell. I would like to find help for him and a support group for me.

The National Alliance for the Mentally Ill receives hundreds of calls like the one above on a daily basis. Since our founding more than 10 years ago, NAMI has become the leading organization for people suffering from mental illness and their families. Our rapid growth, from 256 persons in 1980 to over 130,000 members and 1,008 affiliate groups now, also means that NAMI is one of the fastest growing self-help organizations in the country.

This success can be attributed to a combination of factors, including luck, fortuitous timing and aggressive marketing. NAMI's formation grew out of families' frustration with the "mental health" system, inadequate systems of care for people with these illnesses and the terrible stigma associated with mental illness. Two events in the early 1980's helped to stimulate NAMI growth. First, the self-

Charles R. Harman, MS, is Director of Communications at the National Alliance for the Mentally Ill.

help movement in America proliferated. Second, science made tremendous advances in understanding the human brain and serious mental illnesses such as schizophrenia and manic depression. Dr. Lewis Judd, director of the National Institute of Mental Health from 1987 to 1990 said that 90 percent of all that is known about the brain has been learned in the last 10 years. This information has empowered families to speak out without shame for the first time. As a result, NAMI membership swelled.

NAMI AS A CATALYST

NAMI capitalized on the climate of the '80's by becoming the source of help, hope and action for families of persons suffering from mental illness. This was first accomplished by *reacting* to stigmatizing depictions of mental illness. In 1985, for example, the Hasbro toy company created a doll named, "Zartran: The Paranoid Schizophrenic," and labeled it as "the enemy." NAMI coordinated a letter writing campaign to Hasbro and NAMI leaders were granted a meeting with Hasbro President Alan Hassenfeld. The company apologized, immediately removed the product from the market and funded the creation of a public education/anti-stigma position at NAMI. NAMI was successful in having several other products removed from the market.

Attention was also placed on the media, which had a long history of stereotyping and ridiculing mental illness under the guise of entertainment. NAMI's action in this area included persuading the major television networks to delete or change offensive material. In more than one instance, disclaimer tags were placed at the end of movies containing references to mental illness, offering clarification about what mental illness actually is and referring viewers to NAMI for more information.

Perhaps NAMI's greatest success, however, has been its outreach to the general public. We started with the assumption that most people did not intentionally stigmatize mental illness, rather they simply did not know and did not understand that they were being insensitive.

NAMI took an aggressive marketing approach. We initially focused on gaining national visibility and identity. We placed emphasis on training members to be active marketers in their communities. With "boiler plate" materials and guidance from NAMI, the local volunteers became quite effective in marketing mental illness and their local chapter. The national office focused its efforts on developing materials that could be used by a widely diverse membership—from a handful of members of a local alliance in Minot, North Dakota to 2,000 AMI members of Greater Chicago, which has a paid staff and an office.

BUILDING RELATIONSHIPS
WITH OTHER NATIONAL ORGANIZATIONS

NAMI also developed working relationships at the local and national levels with professional organizations such as the American Psychiatric Association.

NAMI also became active in promotions and the use of media. We successfully aligned ourselves with the television networks and producers who involved us in the production of several high powered made-for-TV movies and documentaries on mental illness. These included Hallmark Hall of Fame's PROMISE, NBC's STRANGE VOICES, and CNN's PEACE OF MIND. Each of these special programs identified NAMI as a source of information and support. STRANGE VOICES, for example, included a scene of actress Valarie Harper attending a local AMI meeting (AMI members were really used!). Co-star Nancy McKeon recorded a public service message about NAMI that was broadcast at the movie's conclusion.

A NATIONAL CAMPAIGN

In 1989, NAMI decided to try for the "big leagues" of promotion by soliciting several New York advertising agencies. Finally, Partners & Shevack, Inc. agreed to create a pro bono campaign for NAMI. The agency treated NAMI like any other client and mental illness like any other product. Since nearly all advertising is based on consumer research, the agency was eager to learn about current public opinion about mental illness. The Robert Wood Johnson Foundation Program for the Chronically Mentally Ill had just finished collecting data for its survey of attitudes about mental illness and, after being approached by NAMI, agreed to share the information with Partners & Shevack. This was extremely helpful, especially since the data was current and available without cost.

Based on the research and discussions with NAMI staff and members, the agency developed the following creative strategy:

I. *Problem the Advertising Must Solve*

Problem
> People are afraid of/fear persons afflicted with mental illnesses.

Objective
> To allay the public's fears of persons afflicted with mental illnesses and create a sympathetic environment towards people with these diseases.

II. *Target Audience*

1. The General Public.
2. Family members of persons afflicted with mental illnesses (use 800 number).

III. *Strategy*

> Confront the public's fear head-on through the use of available facts:
>   • Medication can help control mental illness
>   • Success story—people with mental illnesses can function and succeed in society
>   • Mental illness is an organic brain disease

IV. *Tone and Manner*
> Extremely impactful, highly emotional, shocking.

DEVELOPING PARTNERSHIPS

During the initial meetings with Partners and Shevack, NAMI approached the National Association of Mental Health Information Officers (NAMHIO), a national organization made up of communications directors at community mental health centers, state hospitals, and state departments of mental health. NAMHIO joined NAMI to co-sponsor the project. This arrangement offered NAMI additional exposure and distribution of the campaign materials by professional communicators. It also provided NAMHIO its first opportunity to participate in a public education project on a national level.

With guidance from NAMI and NAMHIO, the agency moved ahead and developed a series of creative drafts. Some of the first drafts were construed as too shocking, but all were very creative. Finally the agency, NAMI and NAMHIO agreed on a creative concept that met the objectives outlined in the creative strategy. Basically, the desire was to show former patients in real life, positive settings. To insure penetration of the message, it was important to make the representations in a creative manner. A campaign slogan, "The Most Shocking Thing About Mental Illness is How Little We Understand It," was developed. The main ad that was developed (see Figure 1) was the result of this effort. The TV spot was extremely creative. It began with the following words, read in a somber voice and flashed across the screen, "WARNING: The following scenes may shock you. They contain graphic depictions of the everyday lives of real people who suffer from serious mental illness." By setting the stage for a "worst case" scenario, the PSA then surprises viewers with three vignettes of positive images of mentally ill people. The first shows Susan, who "suffers from clinical depression," working on a piece of art with her father proudly looking over her work. Next, two men, one of whom has manic depression, are playing a rousing game of basketball. In the third scene, Karen, who suffers from schizophrenia, is shown playing the piano with her little brother sitting beside her. The announcer concludes, "It may come as a shock, but many people with mental illness can lead lives that aren't so different from yours. To understand more, call the National Alliance for the Mentally Ill toll-free 1-800-950-NAMI." While most commercials have actors portraying real life, this PSA used people who were not actors, but who had actually suffered from mental illness.

One of the strongest elements of NAMI's campaign was placement. The print ads and TV PSA were packaged as part of an "Edu-

FIGURE 1

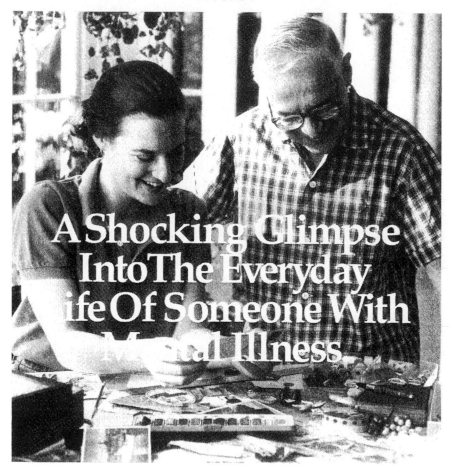

Susan, shown here with her father, does not fit neatly into our preconceptions about people with mental illness. She has a career and is an accomplished artist. And like many Americans who suffer from mental illness, she has responded positively to professional treatment and to the presence, sympathy and *understanding* of friends and family. To understand more about mental illness, or to find help if someone you know suffers from mental illness, contact the National Alliance for the Mentally Ill.

The most shocking thing about mental illness is how little people understand it.

To understand more, call 1-800-950-NAMI.

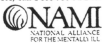

cation Kit'' that included a camera-ready billboard, posters, a fact sheet, letter to the editor, editorial, and clip art (see Figure 2). These materials reinforced the campaign theme. The entire package was made available to members of NAMI and NAMHIO for $25. This restriction on availability encouraged membership in either of the organizations and added value to the memberships.

NAMI placed the ads in the national media. Several national TV networks, including CBS, CNN, WOR, WGN and The Nashville Network aired the PSA. The print ads received excellent pro bono placement, including a full-page ad in US NEWS, a quarter page ad in BETTER HOMES & GARDENS and a quarter page ad in PSY-CHIATRIC NEWS. The combined circulation of these publications was over 7 million and the ad space was valued at $72,264!

NAMI and NAMHIO members were equally successful in placing the materials locally. In West Virginia, for example, the state Alliance for the Mentally Ill persuaded the governor and the first lady to record a special tag at the end of the PSA. Elsewhere, the

FIGURE 2

The most shocking thing about mental illness is how little people understand it.

To understand more,
call 1-800-950-NAMI.

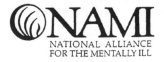

ads and PSA were placed in local newspapers and magazines, on hundreds of local stations, and billboards appeared nationwide.

The campaign was launched during Mental Illness Awareness Week in October 1990. At the same time, NAMI implemented its "HELPLINE" service, a toll-free phone service offering information about mental illness and referral to local NAMI affiliates. The HELPLINE number was included on the advertising materials. NAMI also aggressively promoted the number through the national media. In the first three months the HELPLINE number was included in USA TODAY, PBS "Frontline," ANN LANDERS, READER'S DIGEST, OPRAH WINFREY, LADIES HOME JOURNAL, PARENT'S MAGAZINE, and the ABC movie of the week, "Call Me Anna." This exposure has resulted in thousands of calls to the HELPLINE. During November 1990, 13,875 people called the HELPLINE, talking for a total of 39,383 minutes! "Call Me Anna," the movie about Patty Duke's life and struggle with manic depression, stimulated 7,880 calls in one week alone. Membership recruitment is an integral part of the HELPLINE referral process and NAMI expects a large increase in membership.

Professionals continue to play an integral part of NAMI's marketing strategy and are invited to join as Associate Members. Many local Alliance groups and professionals are already working quite well together.

NAMI's growth is certainly a gauge of successful marketing. Although it is much harder to quantify success in the area of public opinion and the reduction of stigma, NAMI members feel confident that they are changing attitudes. The political climate regarding funding for mental illness research has certainly been bright, with the National Institute of Mental Health receiving record budget increases each of the past three years. While many government agencies were having their 1991 budgets cut, NIMH received a 17 percent increase!

NAMI is clearly meeting a need. We are feeding the hunger for information and support that has long been neglected. NAMI is transforming tremendous pain and personal suffering into energy and action. As our tag line from a previous campaign states, "We're out to change a lot of minds."

EMULATING THE NAMI
MARKETING MODEL

Although certain market conditions and timing can greatly determine the potential success of any marketing effort, planning and persistence helped to insure NAMI's success. The following five recommendations offer some insight into NAMI's efforts.

1. *Think Big:* Define your market in as large an area as possible. Don't be afraid to approach the largest public relations agency seeking pro bono help, or ask the top-rated TV station for a multiple series on mental illness. This approach does not always work, but it usually produces better than average results.
2. *Take Advantage of Opportunities:* Always be on the lookout for ways to include your efforts in events, activities or media coverage that is already planned. For example, if you hear that a prominent mental illness researcher is going to be in your area, ask his or her permission for you to arrange media interviews. Also try to find local "heroes" who can help you tell a story, promote your agenda or even fund important activities. This strategy is cost-effective and generally takes very little time to coordinate. NAMI gained much of its publicity by "tagging on" to activities and media exposure that was already in production. Always have something to offer those who help you, such as a desire to help increase a TV station's ratings, positive media exposure for a local company or an award for a local reporter.
3. *Develop Coalitions:* Simply developing a coalition to fill up your letterhead is worthless. Find a small number of key groups and leaders who are willing to *work* with you. Coalitions will give your effort more credibility, exposure and outreach. Develop a tight agenda and a limited number of activities that your group will undertake so that your coalition is focused. Local NAMI groups should be your first call.
4. *Create One Message:* Have your coalition develop one single message. A single message communicated by several organizations is much more effective than flooding the media with multiple, and perhaps mixed, messages.

5. *Use Multiple Media:* NAMI's message has been successfully placed in the traditional media such as television, newspaper and radio. But we have also taken advantage of non-traditional media, including the Goodyear Blimp, Domino's pizza boxes, restaurant place mats, a clothing outfitter, and Christmas tree ornaments.

CONCLUSION

While NAMI's growth and visibility are certainly signs of its marketing success, it has no desire to rest on its laurels. The key for the organization will be to continue to advance its agenda and outreach in a more sophisticated manner to an even greater number of people. To that end, marketing will maintain its conspicuous presence in the organization and will provide NAMI with a stronger presence in society.

A Marketing Audit
for the Public Mental Health System:
A Review of the Torrey Report

Greg Carlson

SUMMARY. This article examines the *Care of the Seriously Mentally Ill; A Rating of State Programs (1990)* by Torrey, E. Fuller, Karen Erdman, Sidney M. Wolfe, and Laurie M. Flynn, A Joint Publication of Public Citizen Health Research Group and the National Alliance for the Mentally Ill, as a macro-marketing audit of the public mental health system.

INTRODUCTION

In the report entitled, *Care of the Seriously Mentally Ill: A Rating of State Programs*, the authors in conjunction with the National Alliance for the Mentally Ill (NAMI) and the Public Citizen Health Research Group, provide a detailed commentary on the state of the public mental health system in the United States. It's often referred to as the "Torrey" Report because of the senior author. In its third edition, this biannually published document proceeds to systematically rank the 50 states as a "consumer guide" to answer the question, "If I or a family member had a serious mental illness, in what state would that person be most likely to receive good public services?" While the subject matter is certainly more emotional than that contained in other "consumer guides," this document is intended to enlighten consumers, family members, service providers, legislators and other publics of the best and worst mental illness services available to them. In marketing terms, the process the au-

Greg Carlson, MBA, is Director of Planning for the Alabama Department of Mental Health/Mental Retardation in Montgomery, AL.

203

thor utilizes in his quest to rank state mental health systems is very similar to the commonly used marketing audit. According to Philip Kotler (1987), a classical marketing audit in non-profit organizations involves, "a comprehensive, systematic, independent and periodic examination of an organization's [system's] marketing environment, objectives, strategies and activities with a view of determining problem areas and opportunities, and recommending a plan of action to improve the organization's [system's] strategic marketing performance." For more information regarding marketing audits in government and social services, see Crompton, Lamb (1986). Marketing audits are regularly used for organization analysis (for an example of designing a marketing audit for a mental health organization, see Hill (1989)).

These four basic characteristics (comprehensive, systematic, independent and periodic) of a marketing audit are thoroughly addressed in this revealing and very candid report which has effectively raised the consciousness of not only the officials in the public mental health system but also among other publics associated with that system. This report, serves as a "macro-audit" of the entire public mental health system. The conclusions drawn in this marketing audit are substantiated by numerous diagnostic procedures ranging from the more analytical approaches of data collection and analysis to one which is less analytical yet nonetheless impressive—anecdotal individual examples. With respect to the basic underpinnings or functions of the marketing concept, Dr. Torrey's audit incorporates in his deliberations the areas of product, place, price, and promotion.

MAJOR CRISES

The first chapter emphasizes the major crises facing the seriously mentally ill population and is supported by both recent research findings about each crisis as well as anecdotal information. Table 1 provides a listing of these crises.

In this chapter the authors' descriptions of the public mental health system in general seem to parallel those characteristics of a product oriented organization or system that is preoccupied with

TABLE 1. Eight Current Crises

Homelessness - There are more than twice as many people with schizophrenia and manic-depressive psych... living in public shelters and on the streets than there are in public mental health hospitals.

Prison/Jails/Inappropriate Settings - There are more people with schizophrenia and manic-depressive psych... in prisons and jails than in public mental hospitals.

Lack of Treatment - Increasing episodes of violence by seriously mentally ill individuals are a conseque... of not receiving treatment.

Manpower Shortages - Mental health professionals have abandoned the public sector and patients w... serious mental illnesses.

Ineffective Distribution/Providers - Most community mental health centers have been abysmal failures.

Resource Allocation - Funding of public services for individuals with serious mental illness is chaotic.

Management - An undetermined portion of public funds for services to people with serious mental illne... is literally being stolen.

Service Specifications/Guidelines - Guidelines for serving people with mental illnesses are often made at t... the federal and state level by administrators who have had no experience in this field.

producing services which it thinks would be good for the consumers it serves. Despite the fact that its consumers may not be utilizing its service, the product oriented organization still strongly believes in the value of its offerings. The inference in this discussion is the need for a strategic marketing plan which is firmly based upon a consumer orientation wherein the public mental health system should value the tasks of (a) determining the perceptions, needs and wants of its target markets, and (b) satisfying the consumer through the design, pricing, promotion and distribution of appropriate and responsive services. According to the authors, the seriously mentally ill are currently being served, many times by default, in inappropriate distribution systems (i.e., shelters, jails, prisons, and private sector organizations such as community groups, churches, etc.) The system's product/service mix is inadequate and non-responsive to the needs and wants of its target market as evidenced by the number of seriously mentally ill individuals not receiving basic human services (i.e., housing, employment, medical/dental care, etc.). There are sizeable segments of the mental health system's market which are either unserved or underserved.

Questions regarding the optimal allocation of resources both monetary and in terms of qualified personnel to meet the expressed needs of its target markets, remain unanswered. The mission of the system as well as its corresponding strategic marketing objectives are not adequately defined. Due to other more profitable and seemingly more attractive segments of the overall mental health field, the availability of qualified service professionals such as psychiatrists, psychologists, etc., willing to work in the public mental health system remains in short supply. The exchange system on the part of consumers is not perceived as worth the product/service offering of the public mental health system. The product management system is generally viewed as ineffective as well as inefficient to the extreme that public resources are targeted in directions contradictory to the intended wishes of the donors/taxpayers. Finally, the lack of a marketing audit at the individual state level by qualified persons has in many cases prevented the timely resolution of these crises.

IMPROVING THE SYSTEM

Chapter 2 boldly presents six proposals which the authors believe will lead to an improved system of services for the seriously mentally ill population. These six proposals are outlined in Table 2.

First of all, the authors stress that market segmentation must be accomplished and that the mission of the public mental health system must be clearly defined in consumer oriented terms. Target market (population) definitions should reflect this organizational mission. Careful consideration should be given to available resources in satisfying the needs of the stated target population. Likewise, the development of the product/service mix must be carefully designed and coordinated to ensure continuity of the service objectives. The available resources then can be optimally allocated to the major elements of the marketing mix (i.e., quality of service, distribution/accessibility, promotion, and pricing). In implementing this marketing strategy, the system must decide which market segments it should enter, expand, or withdraw from, and then must determine the resource consequences of each decision. The system must also develop pricing (revenue) strategies and objectives—to enhance both product effectiveness and efficiency.

CHARACTERISTICS OF A GOOD SERVICE PLAN

Chapter 4 proceeds to describe what the authors perceive as good services, or in other words, those factors which will enable states to analyze and design a service system (product mix) which is truly consumer oriented. Table 3 summarizes these factors within the categories of (1) hospital services, (2) outpatient and community support services, (3) vocational rehabilitation services, (4) housing services and (5) children's services.

As public organizations mature, their product mix (those services which they offer) often shifts. This certainly appears to be the case with the public mental health system as its philosophy shifts from the more intrusive and restrictive mode of state hospitalization to the less intrusive, less restrictive types of services to enable individ-

TABLE 2. Six Proposals to Improve Services

Market Segmentation - Public mental health programs must serve people with serious mental illness as a priority; if less than 75 percent of a program's resources are going to this group, its state and federal subsidies should be terminated.

Expanded Service Distribution - All psychiatrists, psychologists, and psychiatric social workers should be required to donate, pro bono, one hour of a week of work to public programs. Federal and state supported training programs for such professionals should include an automatic payback obligation.

Qualified Providers - Since psychiatrists have abandoned the public sector, psychologists, physician assistants and nurse practitioners should be given special training and allowed to prescribe psychiatric medication. This program should initially be piloted in three to five states.

Resource Allocation - The chaotic funding of public services for individuals with serious mental illnesses needs a total overhaul.

Mismanagement Resolution - Budgets of public mental health illness programs should be examined for possible theft.

Service Guidelines - All administrators of public programs for people with mental illness should spend at least one-half day each week working with mentally ill people.

TABLE 3. Good Services—Factors to Be Considered

PITAL SERVICES

<u>Quality of Staff</u> -• Credentials/Licenses • Work History • Training •Salaries • Consumer Evaluations
<u>Quantity of Staff</u> - •Optimal Staffing Levels •Overtime/Reassignment •Weekend Staff Ratios
<u>Quality of Treatment</u> - •Individualized Treatment •Medication Monitoring •Extensive Assessments • Patie
Dignity/Respect • Patient Education • Minimal Seclusion/Restraint •Specialized Programs • Case Managem
•Discharge Planning •Legal Rights Protections •Internal Advocacy
<u>Environment</u> - •Privacy •Personal Belongings •Decorative Settings •Individualized Meals •Special Activit
•Natural Clothing •Life Safety Standards

PATIENT/COMMUNITY SUPPORT SERVICES

<u>Quality of Staff</u> - (Same as Hospital Services)
<u>Quantity of Staff</u> - (Same as Hospital Services)
<u>Quality of Treatment</u> - (Same as Hospital Services) - •Case Management •Hospital/Community Agreeme
•Daily Living Assistance •Crisis Services •Psychosocial Rehabilitation •Support Services •Soc
Opportunities•Counseling/Education •Compeer Programs •Income Assistance •Specialized Progra
•Outpatient Commitment •Outreach/Mobile Services •Jail/Prison Outreach •Educated L
Enforcement•Homeless Outreach •Home Health Care •Consumer Employment/Case Managem
•Systematic Evaluation/Monitoring

ATIONAL REHABILITATION

•Availability •Non-time Limited •Pre-vocational Services •Employment Options •Volunteer Progra
•Competitive Employment Alternatives •Supported Employment •Job Development •Job Clubs

TABLE 3 (continued)

NG

•Sufficiency in Public Housing •Housing Options •Independence Goal •Affordable •Geographically Scattered •Safe, Pleasant, Accessible •Flexibility •Privacy •Personal Possessions •Homemaker Services •Respite Housing •Service Accessibility

REN'S SERVICES

General Service Requirements - •Individualized Treatment •Specialized Services •Family Integrity

Hospital Services - •Adequacy of Inpatient Resources •Inpatient Standards •Accredited Educational Opportunities •Family Involvement in Treatment •Family Education and Support

Residential Treatment - •Adequate Residential Opportunities •Homelike and Decorative •Therapeutic Foster Care •Flexibility

Outpatient and Community Support Services - •Specified Training/Certification •Hospital/Community Collaboration •Case Management •Mobile Services •Day Programs •After School/Summer Programs •Emergency/Crisis Services •Home-based Intervention •Counseling and Education •Respite Services •Community Activities •Financial Assistance •Specialized Programs •Outreach Services

Transitional Services - •Specialized Services •Local Interagency Coordination •Independent Living Opportunities •Vocational Services •Educational Support

School System Services - •Teacher Training •Prompt Assessment •Appropriate Treatment •Adequate Services •Mental Health System Coordinators

Juvenile Justice System Services - •Staff Training •Prompt Assessment •Appropriate Treatment •Adequate Services •Mental Health System Coordinators

Intra-agency Coordination - •Local Interagency Coordination •Case Management Involvement •Resource Allocation uals with serious mental illness to live as independently as possible within the community. According to the authors, the agency that ultimately provides these needed services is, "from the point of view of a person with a serious mental illness . . . inconsequential; she or he wants the needed services to be delivered and does not care how they are organized as long as they meet minimally acceptable standards." The boundaries therefore, by which the needed services are governed and delivered, need not be restricted by that which has been traditional. New and innovative approaches targeted toward satisfying and maintaining consumers in their community are essential in the process of converting from the historic product oriented system to one which is truly consumer oriented and consumer responsive.

RANKINGS OF STATES

Chapter 5 presents the methodological approach by which Dr. Torrey ranks the states. He is quick to note that even the best of state public mental health programs have a long way to go toward achieving the ideal service system. The number one ranked state's score was still just 68% of a possible 100. Table 4 provides an overview of the factors which tend to relate to good programs.

CONCLUSION

This report can serve the state public mental health systems well if a consumer oriented management philosophy is carefully introduced in the planning and product/service development process. The strategic marketing plan concept is not new and is embodied in the underlying principles and philosophies associated with federal legislation found in Public Law 99-660 which mandates a planning process incorporating all relevant publics. The political and entrenched practices of tradition in any organization, but particularly in the public mental health agency can, however, effectively neutralize meaningful changes from the historic product orientation to a consumer orientation. Thus, those phenomena associated with organizational change must also be considered and addressed in the

TABLE 4. Factors Related to Good Programs

APITA SPENDING

Higher per capita income spending on mental health services was found to be associated with the better performing (ranking) states. Strong correlation exists between per capita expenditure and its score c vocational rehabilitation, housing, and children's services.

RAPHY

There are strong regional influences on the quality of services to people with serious mental illness. This largely accounted for by their respective funding levels.

: MENTAL HEALTH DIRECTOR's EXPERIENCE

Higher expenditures on mental health services tend to be associated with those states which have director with the greatest experience.

N SERVICES SPENDING

A state's per capita spending on mental health services is associated with the overall level of human service expenditures.

D

The level of HUD funding is not a predictor of better housing for the seriously mentally ill.

:NDING/POPULATION FACTORS

Scores on children services scores seemed to be related to both the state's education spending and its me health per capita expenditures.

'CHOLIGIST DENSITY

No relationship exists between the state's inpatient and outpatient services and the state's concentratic psychologists.

CIAL WORKER DENSITY

A higher per capita social worker ratio did not result in better rankings.

TIONAL ALLIANCE FOR THE MENTALLY ILL MEMBERSHIP (NAMI)

Motivating citizen involvement as measured by AMI member concentration is related to the cost and qu of state mental health programs.

utilization of the "Torrey Report" factors for a successful and meaningful strategic marketing in the public mental health sector.

REFERENCES

Crompton, John L., Charles W. Lamb, Jr., (1986); *Marketing Government and Social Services*, pp. 75-109, New York: John Wiley and Sons.
Hill, C. Jeane (1989). The Challenge of Auditing Mental Health, *Journal of Marketing for Mental Health*, 2(1), 17-25.
Kotler, Philip, Alan R. Andreasen (1987). *Strategic Marketing For Non-Profit Organizations*. p. 638, Englewood Cliffs, New Jersey: Prentice-Hall, Inc.

Printed and bound by CPI Group (UK) Ltd, Croydon, CR0 4YY

22/10/2024

01777623-0006